Foreword

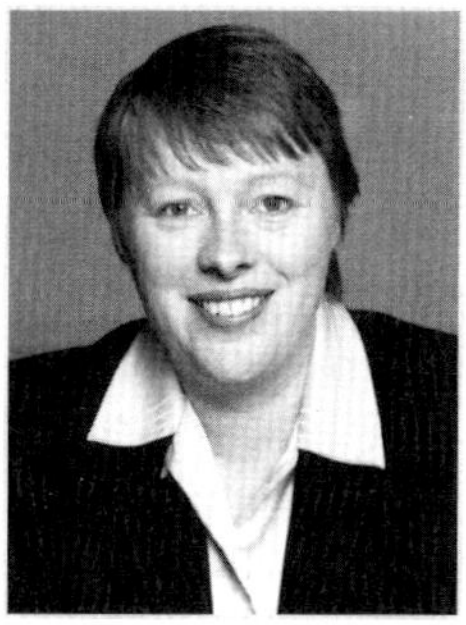

Legislative change since the last edition of this *Buildings for all to use*, published in 1996, reflects the increasing value society places on ensuring everyone is treated fairly. The introduction of Part 3 of the Disability Discrimination Act (DDA), which affects service providers and the Special Educational Needs and Disability Act 2001 which brought access to education within the remit of the DDA, highlight that accessibility and inclusion should be key considerations for service providers, employers and organisations providing education and training. It makes good business sense to make services and facilities accessible for disabled people and increased accessibility will enable the UK economy to benefit from the considerable spending power of disabled people and their friends and families.

Existing buildings present many constraints and challenges. This guide gives strategic and detailed design guidance on how to overcome them. An inclusive approach to the built environment will result in better buildings for everyone. We know that good access provision can help parents with pushchairs, people carrying shopping and older people, but even the best designed building needs proactive and ongoing management to ensure it remains accessible to all. A little thought and creativity can make a big difference.

I welcome this new edition of *Buildings for all to use*, because it will help those concerned with policy, management and design decisions to identify every available opportunity to improve acccssibility.

Maria Eagle

Maria Eagle,
Minister for Disabled People

April 2004

Acknowledgements

Research contractor
Research Group for Inclusive Environments,The University of Reading. (www.reading.ac.uk/ie)

Lead authors
Professor Keith Bright MSc FRICS FBEng MCIOB NRAC, is Director of Keith Bright Consultants Ltd and Professor of Inclusive Environments at The University of Reading. He is a chartered building surveyor, consultant member of the National Register of Access Consultants and a member of its management committee. He is a recognised national and international expert in the design and management of inclusive, accessible environments.

Susan Flanagan BSc MSc MRICS, is a chartered surveyor who has worked in both the private and the public sector. She joined RGIE in 1996 after completing an MSc in Information Technology from the University of the West of England at Bristol. Susan is an experienced access auditor and has worked on several research projects including the use of colour and contrast in the built environment, wayfinding in public buildings and the use of assistive technology in the existing homes of older people.

Co-authors
Justine Embleton MSc Dip COT NRAC, is a registered access consultant and an occupational therapist. She gained an MSc in Inclusive Environments from the University of Reading in 2002 and has worked for the last three years as education manager in RGIE. Justine is a regular speaker on issues related to accessibility and the DDA and, through Embleton Consultancy, also operates as an independent access consultant.

Laura Selbekk MSc NRAC, is a consultant member of the National Register of Access Consultants and an assessor for the Register. She has worked as an access officer and access consultant in Surrey since 1996 and in 2003 gained an MSc in Inclusive Environments at The University of Reading. Laura also works as an independent access consultant. She has considerable experience in matters associated with the DDA and, as a trainer licensed by the Disability Rights Commission, is a regular speaker nationally.

Author of Chapter 13
Dr Geoffrey Cook BSc PhD CEng FCIOB MCIBSE MSLL MIESNA, is an experienced leader of research projects in lighting, colour and low vision. He has published widely and is acknowledged both nationally and internationally as a leading expert in these areas. Geoff is a member of several national and international committees related to research into lighting and low vision and is Director of the Research Group for Inclusive Environments at The University of Reading.

Authors of case studies 7.1 and 7.2
Tom Lister, Margaret Macleish, David Frogatt, Buro Happold Disability Design Consultancy
www.burohappold.com

The following photographs and figures are reproduced with permission of:

Buro Happold Disability Design Consultancy:	7.1–7.3 and Figures 7a & 7b
David Barbour/Building Design Partnership Ltd:	7.4–7.6, 7.8, 7.11–7.13
Dorma UK:	6.2, 6.3, 9.10, 9.15–9.17, 9.22, 9.23, 14.20
Jason Randall:	7.7, 7.9, 7.10, 7.14, 7.15
RNIB:	2.1–2.4.

Following CIRIA's usual practice, the research project was guided by a Steering Group which comprised:

Chair

Andrew McLeish	WS Atkins

Members

Simon Chapman	Dorma UK
Ted Finneron	Representative of the Automatic Door Suppliers Association
David Heath	English Heritage
Bob Hellis	Lewisham Borough Council
Yvonne Howard	Transport for London
Peter Wright	Transport for London
Mairi Johnson	Commission for Architecture in the Built Environment (CABE)
Katherine Phipps	JMU Access Partnership
Malcolm Potter	DTI representative, Davis Langdon Consultancy
David Pickles	English Heritage
Peter Roe	Representative of the Construction Industry Council, AE Thornton-Firkin and Partrners
Andrew Shipley	Disability Rights Commission
Neil Smith	Centre for Accessible Environments

CIRIA's research manager for the project was Sarah Reid.

Project funders

The project was funded by: DTI Partners in Innovation
CIRIA Core members
Dorma UK
Phlexicare
Automatic Door Suppliers Association
Rediweld Rubber & Plastic

Contributors

CIRIA and the authors are grateful for all the help given to this project by the funders, the members of the steering group, and by the many organisations and individuals who were consulted, and who provided information. In particular, the contributions of the following individuals are acknowledged:

David Petherick	observer from the Office of the Deputy Prime Minister
Professor Peter Barker	Disabled Persons Transport Advisory Committee (DPTAC)
Mr John Miller	John Miller Partnership
Mrs Janet Parker	Parker Knight Associates
Dr Monnica Stewart	Re: St Mary's Church, Kintbury
Mr Tim Smith	West Berks Council

Contributions do not imply that individual funders, contributors or steering group members necessarily endorse all views expressed in the published book.

British Library Cataloguing in Publication Data

A catalogue record is available for this book from the British Library.

Published by CIRIA, Classic House, 174–180 Old Street, London EC1V 9BP, UK.

CIRIA C610

Contents

List of tables

List of figures

Photographs

Abbreviations

affl	above finished floor level
ATM	Automated Teller Machine
BSI	British Standards Institution
CIBSE	Chartered Institute of Building Services Engineers
CIE	Commission Internationale de l'Éclairage
ODPM	Office of the Deputy Prime Minister
DfT	Department for Transport
ICEL	International Committee for Emergency Lighting
SLL	Society of Light and Lighting.

Part one – background and general principles

1 Introduction

1.1 The aim of this book

An environment that is inclusive and accessible will allow all users to participate independently and equally, according to their ability. Therefore, in designing and managing an accessible environment, it is important to consider how the abilities of users, rather than their disabilities, can be addressed to widen participation.

In modern life there are, for many people, a considerable number of opportunities to buy goods and services, to enjoy employment opportunities in a multitude of professions, to enjoy the benefits of education or to travel great distances. For some, however, such opportunities are very much dependent upon the accessibility of the environments in which the activities are housed. An apparently small issue, such as a single step along a route, an inaccessible ticket machine, inconsistent signage or poor management practices, can present a barrier to some people, preventing them from participating in everyday activities that others take for granted.

In designing a new environment or managing an existing one, it may appear that the apparently diverse needs of disabled and non-disabled users are too difficult to address. However, for many people, the basic needs in using an environment will often be similar, as will the solutions to any problems they experience. For example, a wider door may be incorporated to improve accessibility for a wheelchair user, but a person using a different mobility aid, such as a guide dog or crutches, or someone pushing a buggy or carrying luggage, would also benefit from wider doors. Similarly, providing a level entrance or appropriate signage, essential for many disabled people, will not disadvantage other users. Indeed, in most cases it will enhance usability for everyone.

Those who offer services to members of the public, or who employ others, are now obliged by legislation to ensure that those services are accessible to all and that employment arrangements do not place disabled people at a disadvantage. For some this can present difficulties, not least because the physical nature of the buildings or environments they currently use can make it difficult to ensure equality of access.

A service provider can be anyone who offers a service to the public, either free or for payment. This is a broad group but would include, for example, hotels, guest houses, shops, pubs, restaurants, banks, building societies, hospitals, surgeries, bus and rail stations, theatres, cinemas, libraries, museums, courts, central and local government services, and churches. For employers, legislation currently relates to those organisations with 15 or more employees, but from October 2004 it encompasses all employers.

In reality, many of the buildings that service providers, employers and most of us will use for many years to come, already exist. Many of the buildings now being constructed are designed around philosophies and accessibility standards that are now out of date, yet the service provider or the employer must, by law, operate around any shortcomings in the buildings they use to ensure discrimination does not occur.

While it is important to ensure that all new buildings meet appropriate accessibility standards, the more pressing need for many is to consider how existing buildings, environments and management practices can be adapted to meet the requirements of the legislation.

The aim of this book, as of its predecessor, is to examine the complex area of making existing environments accessible, and to offer practical advice on the alterations that can be made, in terms of physical features and management practices, to maximise accessibility for everyone.

1.2 The content

Although this book is primarily a design guide, it is not solely for designers. In the provision and management of the modern built environment there are many individuals, who have a direct influence on its accessibility, either in the provision of services or in the opportunities made available for both disabled and non-disabled people. As well as designers, these include owners, managers and users, all of whom will be affected by different obligations, responsibilities and expectations. There are also several areas covered within this book that relate to management practices and legislation, and which will be of particular interest to all "players".

The decision to improve the accessibility of a building or environment may be taken for commercial reasons, in response to lobbying or legislation, to increase the availability of the workforce, or from a management desire to improve the basis on which services or employment opportunities are offered. Very often, the initiator of improvements will not be the designer but the building owner, the developer, the manager of the environment, the disabled users or those supporting them, such as occupational therapists.

It is critical that improvements should be considered in the much wider context of raising standards of accessibility for everyone, something that will obviously benefit both disabled and non-disabled people. This book:

- identifies the main issues affecting accessibility and inclusion
- offers practical and pragmatic guidance
- considers those areas in existing buildings where management practices and procedures working in harmony with physical changes can overcome difficult obstacles
- gives advice on how good management can reduce, or even exclude, additional costs.

Current guidance and indicators of minimum standards generally revolve around BS8300: 2001 and the Approved Document (AD) to Part M of the Building Regulations, revised in 2003 and effective in April 2004. The information contained in BS8300: 2001 is advisory, although it will almost certainly be taken as an indicator of the type of physical changes that would be reasonable to expect when judging the accessibility of an existing building.

In general terms, the AD to Part M is more relevant to new buildings, major refurbishments or changes to those parts of an existing building which offer the main access to a new building or extension. It also covers material alterations, which could, in some cases, be as simple as changing the size of a lobby or the design of a feature previously approved under Part M, such as the design of a door handle or the door itself.

For the purposes of this book, BS8300: 2001, which is more relevant to existing buildings, has been used as the main source to formulate design guidance. Where there are differences in the guidance of BS and the 2004 version of the AD to Part M that may significantly affect potential alterations for an existing building, these have been highlighted.

However, anyone considering alterations to an existing building is advised to consult the 2004 AD to Part M to identify any issues that may relate to new building work, substantial alterations or material alterations and which may affect any physical or managerial changes being proposed.

1.3 The structure

The book is structured in two parts. Part One considers those areas which represent a background of understanding that everyone involved in the design and management of the built environment should have. These include the:

- needs of users
- legislation which has driven changes in the way services, employment opportunities, education and transport facilities are being offered and delivered
- areas that modern management strategies should address
- ways in which addressing inclusion and accessibility may impinge on historic buildings and monuments.

Part One also describes four case studies that demonstrate what can be achieved with careful thought and a willingness to compromise.

Part Two examines in detail the issues associated with improving the physical accessibility of environments. It offers advice on how alterations and management practices can work together to overcome the more difficult access issues that will be found when considering the use of existing buildings. The Appendices offer a comprehensive source of information, guidance and references to complement the main text.

1.4 Features to support the text

1.4.1 Photographs

Photographs, some of which include a green tick ✓ for good practice or a red cross ✗ for issues that fall below acceptable practice, support the text.

The presence of a ✓ or a ✗ does not suggest that everything in the photograph is acceptable or unacceptable. It is used as an indicator of the area being considered, or as a general indicator of practice. Symbols are not used on photographs illustrating general, rather than specific, points.

1.4.2 Cross-referencing

Information is given in the text where it is most appropriate. For example, general guidance is given on doors in Chapter 9 – Entrances, but information is also given in Chapter 11 – Horizontal circulation. Cross-references to relevant paragraph numbers are shown in the box with a blue border at the end of some individual paragraphs (see example).

See 4.3.4, 14.2.1

In a book of this complexity, it is not possible to identify all cross-references throughout the text. Therefore, the ones identified represent the views of the authors on the links that would be most useful to the reader.

2 User needs

2.1 Inclusion

Historically, design guidance on creating new environments or adapting existing ones during refurbishments or repairs, has been largely based around the needs and views of a notional average user. In reality, the needs and abilities of most people, whether disabled or non-disabled, do not match those of this person.

For example, the distances people may be able to travel, either walking or with mobility aids such as wheelchairs, varies, as does the effectiveness of other assistance aids such as spectacles or hearing aids.

Users are generally considered as being "disabled" or "non-disabled" and, because the requirements of disabled people seem to vary, some believe it is impossible to address all of their needs when designing and managing environments. However, there are also many differences in the characteristics of non-disabled people, for example, strength, height, dexterity, stamina, intellectual ability, visual performance, hearing ability or continence.

An inclusive approach to the design of environments accepts that all users have a range of needs and abilities and that these should be addressed by designs that allow the majority of people to use environments comfortably, as independently as possible and, most importantly, safely.

Designing for inclusion does not suggest that there will be no specific areas where additional assistance will be required to meet the needs of some users, for example, providing induction loops to enhance communication for hearing aid users, and tactile surfaces or Braille to assist communication with users who have a visual impairment. However, there is a need to consider such assistance as being supplementary to, and not a replacement for, the provision of good initial design and on-going management of an environment.

2.2 The need

Recent government estimates suggest that there around 9 million disabled adults in the UK, constituting 15 per cent of the electorate. Seven per cent of adults are born with an impairment. The likelihood of developing an impairment increases as people get older, and ranges from approximately five per cent of people under 25 years of age to more than 80 per cent of people of 80 years of age or more. But even though the incidence of disability increases with age, it is wrong to assume that all older people are disabled.

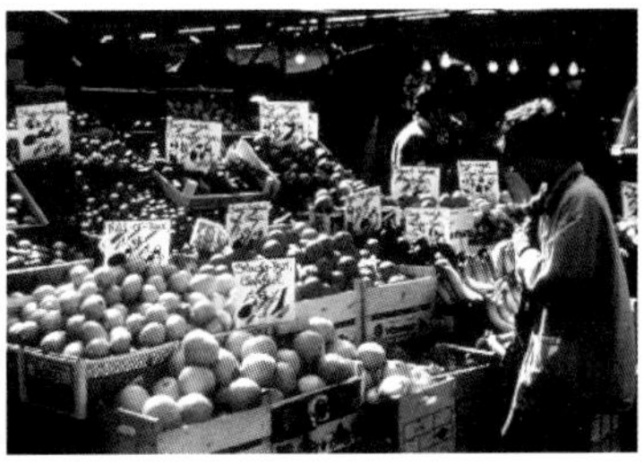

1. A market scene, as seen ... by someone who is fully sighted

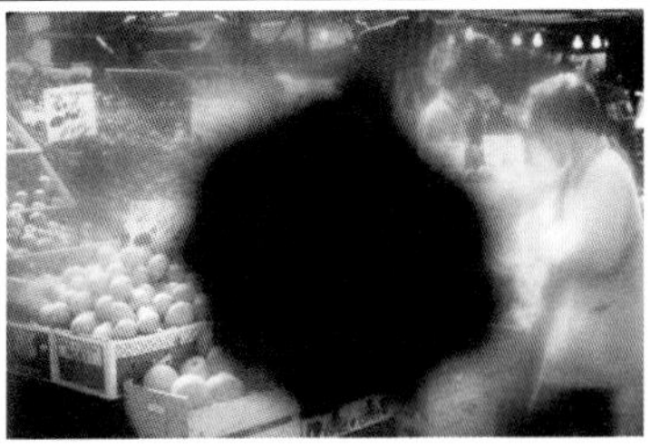

2 ... by someone with central visual field loss

In the UK, there are approximately 600 000 wheelchair users, half of whom use their wheelchairs on a permanent basis. The other half will mainly use their wheelchairs to assist long distance mobility and may be able to undertake certain tasks without using their chair. These tasks might include climbing one or two steps, standing at a urinal (if the correct grab bars are provided), or standing to transfer onto a seat or onto a hotel bed.

There are about 2.5 to 3 million people in the UK with a visual impairment or poor vision. About 1.5 million are registered or could be registered as blind or partially-sighted and are therefore covered by the Disability Discrimination Act 1995.

Of this blind and partially sighted population, 82 per cent have some residual vision which, if maximised, could considerably enhance their ability to gather information and increase their independence. Of the remaining 18 per cent, 14 per cent will have some light perception but will have insufficient vision to make use of, for example, colour and luminance contrast. Only around four per cent of the blind and partially-sighted population see nothing at all. Most of these people will have been blind since birth.

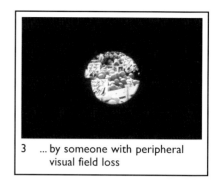

3 ... by someone with peripheral visual field loss

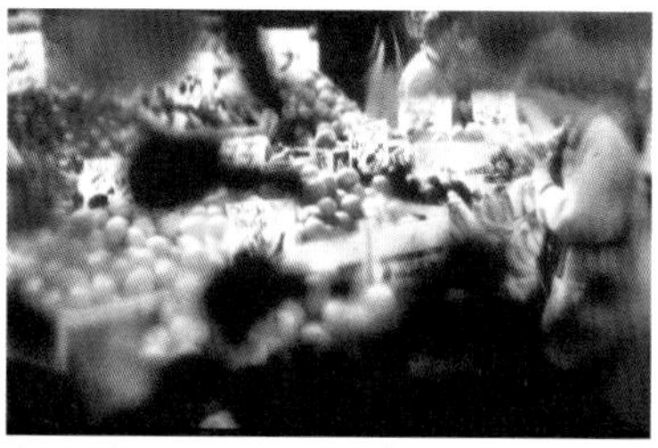
4 ... by someone with general visual field loss

According to the RNID, about 8.7 million people in the UK experience some form of hearing loss. The degree of deafness ranges from mild hearing loss (where there is a problem in following speech), moderate hearing loss (where a hearing aid is commonly used), severe hearing loss (where a hearing aid is of little use) and profound deafness (where there is a complete loss of hearing). About seven per cent of the population are affected by a condition known as Tinnitus, which presents a ringing or buzzing in the ears that can eliminate other sounds which unaffected people take for granted. This may include, for example, audible warnings, recorded messages or answerphones. Many deaf people place great reliance on visual aids such as signs.

For hearing aid users, induction loops, which can be installed easily and at minimal cost, can considerably assist the well-being and participation of a person with a hearing impairment in the workplace, at conferences, job interviews and at all places in the built environment where audible communication is needed.

It is estimated that of the 8.7 million people who experience some loss of hearing, only around a quarter wear hearing aids and, of those, not all will use hearing aids that can be used with an induction loop. For these people (perhaps as many as seven million people), the ability of the people they are communicating with to speak clearly, to have at least a basic understanding of a sign language (such as British Sign Language), to have access to information in readily understandable formats and experience the appropriate use of colour, contrast and lighting, can be critical.

2.3 Models of disability

The label "disabled" is often applied to people whose abilities are considered to fall outside the scope of what some people might suggest are "normal" abilities. At the design stage, it is often assumed that users will fall into one of two categories. One is that of an "able-bodied" young person, fit and with the strength of a young male, unburdened by the need to carry additional goods or equipment and who is blessed with perfection in vision, hearing, manual dexterity. This user also has the intellectual ability to understand misleading information at a glance, will find and interpret inconveniently placed signage and, of course, is right handed. The other category is that of a "disabled" person who is identical to their able bodied counterpart, but is now sitting down. In reality, neither of these categories represents the majority of the users of environments.

An environment should be designed and managed to meet the needs of all the people who will use it – even if their abilities vary. For example, if doorways in a building are of a standard that is too narrow for a wheelchair user, they may be made wider as a "special" provision or to meet a special need of the disabled user. However, someone pushing a pram or carrying luggage, temporarily using crutches, with an assistance dog or simply laden with shopping, would all benefit from the provision of wider doorways.

Similarly, the apparent "special" needs of disabled people are addressed, even in new buildings, by the provision of a ramp to overcome the obstruction of steps. The question is whether the steps were necessary in the first place. A positive user-driven approach to issues such as this, would, in many cases, eliminate any need to undertake "special" adaptations.

2.3.1 The medical model

The medical model of disability suggests a loss of faculty as the principal indicator of the presence of a disability. Sometimes, the medical approach is termed the "personal tragedy approach" where disability is believed to be an unfortunate twist of fate, to be dealt with by individual and largely medically-based interventions. It leads to the assumption that the disabled person is unavoidably dependent on others and that some care is needed in almost everything they do.

2.3.2 The social model

The social model of disability recognises that disability is not only the result of an individual impairment, but is also greatly influenced by the environments that people have to use. These environments were not designed and are often not managed to enable participation by disabled people. The social model recognises that beyond equal opportunity or equal treatment, discrimination has to embrace the principle of equal environmental opportunity, to enable disabled people to access the same opportunities as those available to non-disabled people.

In the social model, a disability is not simply the result of having an impairment but is actually caused, and most certainly accentuated, by society not meeting the needs of people who use environments. The restrictions and barriers experienced by disabled people with impairments can be removed by careful design and management.

2.4 The demand

2.4.1 Awareness

"Visual impairment" is not the same as "blindness." A visually impaired person is someone who is registered or eligible for registration as blind or partially sighted. Around one in 25 of visually impaired people see nothing at all. While some people will be able to discern only changes in lightness/darkness, more than 80 per cent of people with a visual impairment have some residual vision that, if accompanied by appropriate design provision of facilities, can considerably enhance their ability to move around environments and identify features independently and safely.

Although some people may experience difficulties with both communication and understanding, this is not the case in the vast majority of situations, so a person who has difficulty communicating does not, by implication, have an equal difficulty in understanding.

For people who use lip reading as a means of enhancing communication, excessive lip movement and slow speech will only hinder the process. What is needed is clear lip speaking at appropriate (usually standard pace) and for lips to be clearly visible (not hidden by facial hair or hands). Speaking louder is unlikely to help most people, and may well cause unnecessary embarrassment to all concerned. For someone who has lost particular frequencies or ranges of hearing, shouting will not help. If problems occur, the wording being used should be changed. For example, if "Please take a seat" causes difficulty, this could be replaced with "Wait over there please", which may fall more readily within the hearing ability of the person.

It is often suggested that there are not many disabled people and that they do not represent a significant market for goods and services.

It is estimated by the Disability Rights Commission that there are 8.6 million disabled people in the UK who will be covered by the duties imposed on employers and service providers by the Disability Discrimination Act 1995.

However, even one person who is unable to enjoy equal employment opportunities or participate equally in a service being offered, may have redress under the DDA, so the numbers game is largely irrelevant.

2.4.2 The meaning of "disability"

It is not always possible to rely upon visual information or clues to identify what assistance a disabled person might require. The concept of disability as defined in the Disability Discrimination Act 1995 (see also Chapter 3) is extremely wide and goes well beyond the traditional view that a disabled person can be identified by a wheelchair or a guide dog. Under the DDA, an "impairment" is a term which covers both physical and mental impairments and also those sensory or cognition impairments which affect vision, hearing, learning or behaviour.

However, for someone with an impairment to be covered by the Act, it must:

- "be long term" – this includes an impairment which has lasted or is likely to last more than 12 months, or is one which will last for the rest of the life of the person – a terminal illness for example
- affect the person's ability to carry out the type of normal day-to-day activities that are carried out by most people on a regular basis. These activities may involve one or more of 10 categories which comprise mobility, manual dexterity, physical coordination, continence, the ability to lift, carry or move ordinary objects, speech, hearing or eyesight, memory or ability to concentrate, learn or understand, the ability to recognise physical danger.

With the sole exception of glasses or contact lenses, any treatment or equipment that assists, alleviates or removes the effect of the impairment is ignored in considering if a person has an impairment that brings them within the scope of the DDA. A person with a severe disfigurement would be covered by the DDA, without any need for him or her to demonstrate that the impairment has a substantial adverse effect on their ability to carry out normal day to day activities.

2.4.3 The ageing population

The United Kingdom currently has a balanced age population in which the proportion of older people (those over pensionable age) is almost identical to those below pension age. However, within the older population itself the proportion of people over 80 years of age is increasing, and this trend is similar across Europe, the US, Japan and Australasia.

The number of people over pensionable age in the UK is expected to increase from just fewer than 11 million in 2001 to more than 12 million in 2011. The number is expected to peak in 2040 at over 15 million out of a total population of 64 million people, or more than 25 per cent.

In 2001, there were just over one million more children aged under 16 than there were people of state pensionable age. By 2007, the population of state pensionable age is expected to exceed the number of children, and by 2026 is expected to exceed it by nearly two million.

It would be wrong to suggest that all older people have impairments, but it is clear that the demand for accessible, more useable environments will grow as the numbers of older people increase. The year 2040 may seem some way off, but it is well within the age expectancy of many public access buildings currently in existence or about to be constructed.

3 Legislation

3.1 Introduction

This chapter will consider the legislation, regulations and standards relevant to accessibility, disability and inclusion.

Since the 1990s there have been several pieces of new legislation, and alterations made to other existing legislation, that affect the design and management of inclusive, accessible environments. The introduction of the Disability Discrimination Act 1995 (DDA 1995), which became effective in October 1996, has had a major influence on accessibility, both in terms of the physical environment, and in the way that service providers and employers offer, maintain and manage their services and employment opportunities. Major changes in the Building Regulations will also have a major impact on the provision of new and refurbished premises. Advisory codes, such as BS 8300: 2001, are now offering the type of advice that will assist in making decisions about what may constitute "reasonableness" and "acceptability" under the DDA.

3.2 The Disability Discrimination Act 1995

The Disability Discrimination Act 1995 (DDA) introduced new legislation and measures to address discrimination against disabled people and to give them rights in the areas of:

- access to goods, facilities and services
- buying or renting land or property
- employment.

The DDA is civil rights legislation and does not directly require buildings to be accessible to all disabled people and it does not include standards for accessible building design. The main concern of the Act is the service or the employment opportunity within the building. In that respect the DDA covers people not buildings.

Sections of the Act also allow the government to set access standards for public transport, and the provision and delivery of education for disabled pupils and students. The Special Educational Needs and Disability Act 2001 (SENDA) amends and extends sections of the DDA to include duties for disabled pupils and students. The duties imposed by the SENDA amendments are identified in more detail later in 3.2.4 and 3.3.

See 2.4.1, 2.4.2, 3.1, 4.1

3.2.1 The meaning of "discrimination"

"Discrimination" occurs when a disabled person is treated less favourably than a non-disabled person for a reason relating to their disability, and without justification.

3.2.2 Part II – Employment

Under the DDA, it is unlawful for employers to discriminate against disabled people when they apply for a job or in their employment. This includes arrangements and procedures for gaining employment, such as advertisements for employment, application forms, interview arrangements, terms of employment, promotion or training opportunities. Most employers have a duty to make "reasonable adjustments" if a physical feature of their premises, or practices and procedures they adopt, cause a substantial disadvantage to a disabled employee or applicant. The duty on the employer is, "to take such steps as it is reasonable for him to have to take in all the circumstances of the situation", to prevent the disadvantage.

Failure to make reasonable adjustment without an acceptable justification will be construed as discrimination under the Act. There is currently no duty under Part II on an employer with fewer than 15 employees. However, this is highly likely to change October 2004 (see 3.11).

3.2.3 Part III – Access to goods, facilities and services

Part III of the DDA is based on the principle that disabled people should not be treated less favourably, simply because of their impairment, by those who provide goods, facilities and services to the public. Part III applies to any person or organisation that provides a service to the public or a section of the public.

Service providers include hotels, guest houses, shops, pubs, restaurants, banks, building societies, hospitals, surgeries, bus and rail stations, theatres, cinemas, libraries, museums, courts, central and local government services, and churches.

It applies equally to both owner-occupiers and tenants and to services provided with or without payment. Part III of the Act does not cover the manufacture and design of products, as this does not involve the provision of services directly to the public.

From October 1999, service providers have been required to make reasonable adjustments to allow a disabled person to use a service on an equal basis. The duty is being implemented in two stages. The first stage, which took effect in October 1999, required service providers to take reasonable steps to make reasonable adjustments to their policies, practices and procedures which exclude disabled people; to provide auxiliary aids, such as temporary ramps, audio tapes etc; and to find a reasonable alternative method of delivering the service if there is a physical feature which makes it impossible or unreasonably difficult for disabled people to use it.

From October 2004, service providers will have a duty to take such steps "as are reasonable in all the circumstances of the case" to modify physical barriers if they make it impossible or unreasonably difficult for a disabled person to use the service. The steps that service providers must take should meet one of the following four options, which should have been considered and acted upon by October 2004:

1. Remove the feature causing the barrier.
2. Alter the feature so that it no longer has the effect of making it impossible or unreasonably difficult for the disabled person to use the service.
3. Provide a means of avoiding the feature.
4. Make the service available to disabled people by a reasonably alternative method.

3.2.4 Part IV – Education

Part IV of the DDA relates to the provision of education and requires educational establishments in England and Wales to inform parents, students and pupils about the facilities and arrangements available at their institutions to meet the needs of disabled people. Since January 1997, the governing bodies of all maintained schools, except for schools provided solely for students with special needs education, have been required to publish details in their annual reports of the following:

- a description of the admission arrangements for disabled students or pupils
- details of the steps taken to prevent disabled pupils from being treated less favourably than non-disabled pupils
- details of any facilities which are provided to assist access for disabled pupils to their school.

Other duties are also placed on both the Further and the Higher Education Funding Councils.

Publicly-funded education was originally excluded from the provisions of Part III of the DDA (goods, facilities and services), but this exemption was effectively removed by the Special Educational Needs and Disability Act 2001 (SENDA) which came into force in September 2002.

3.2.5 Reasonableness

Under the DDA there are duties on the providers of services, employment and education to take "reasonable" steps to eliminate discrimination. "Reasonableness" must be considered in "all the circumstances of the case" and will almost certainly vary between different situations. The factors about the provider that will be used to determine "reasonableness" include:

- the type of service or opportunity being provided
- the nature of the provider in terms of size and resources
- the effect of the disability on the individual disabled person.

Some of the factors that may be taken into account when considering what is reasonable include:

- whether taking any particular steps will be effective in overcoming the difficulty faced by the disabled person
- the extent to which it is practicable to take the steps
- the financial and other costs of making the adjustment
- the extent of any disruption which would occur when taking the steps
- the extent of the provider's financial and other resources
- the amount of any resources already spent on making adjustments
- the availability of financial or other assistance.

There is no exception for small businesses but, clearly, what would be considered reasonable for a small company or employer may well be different from that considered reasonable for a larger company, even when trying to solve an identical accessibility issue.

The DDA expressly states that a service provider "is not required to take any steps that would fundamentally alter the nature of the service in question, or his trade, profession, or business, or prevent the service from being provided to everyone else".

For employers, the cost of undertaking alteration work for new and existing disabled employees to assist them in the workplace, may be covered, either in full or in part, by government schemes such as Access to Work (operated by local Job Centres).

3.2.6 Sanctions

Actions taken under the DDA are civil proceedings. The DDA does not create any criminal offences but it is a criminal offence to impersonate a disabled person in order to receive preferential treatment under the Act.

A disabled person who believes that discrimination has occurred can bring civil proceedings in either:

- an employment tribunal for claims under Part II (Employment) of the Act
- a county court for claims under Part III (Provision of Goods, Facilities and Services etc) or Part IV (Publicly Funded Education) of the Act.

A disabled person who is successful in an action may be awarded compensation for financial loss, including punitive damages for injury to feelings. Powers reside with the court to prevent the discrimination recurring, perhaps by the use of an injunction, and for use in employment disputes.

3.2.7 Codes of practice

A code of practice, which uses worked examples to illustrate how compliance with the duties imposed by the Act might be met, supports each part of the DDA. Codes do not impose legal obligations and are not authoritative statements of law. However, they may be used as evidence in legal proceedings.

One code of practice for "The Elimination of Discrimination in the Field of Employment against Disabled Persons or Persons who have a Disability", gives guidance to employers on the implications of Part II of the Act. It is available from www.disability.gov.uk/dda

3.3 Special Educational Needs and Disability Act 2001

The Special Educational Needs and Disability Act 2001 (SENDA), amended Part IV of the DDA and expanded the duties relating to disabled pupils and students. It also removed the exemption of publicly-funded education from Part III of the Act although, where a duty under Part IV (Education) applies, Part III cannot apply.

Education providers are now required to make reasonable adjustments for disabled students and pupils. The duties include all areas of education, schools, colleges, universities, adult education and youth services, and include a duty:

- not to treat disabled students or pupils less favourably than non-disabled students or pupils without justification
- to make reasonable adjustments to policies, practices and procedures that may discriminate against disabled students or pupils
- to provide education by a "reasonable alternative means" where a physical feature places a disabled student/pupil at a substantial disadvantage
- on local education authorities in England and Wales to plan strategically and increase the overall accessibility to school premises and the curriculum.

Additional duties are placed on the education of post-16 years of age pupils and students in that:

- from September 2002 a duty was imposed not to discriminate against existing and prospective disabled students by treating them less favourably in the provision of student services
- from September 2003 there is a duty to make reasonable adjustments to provide auxiliary aids
- from September 2005 there will be a duty to make adjustments to physical features. This is an anticipatory and continuing duty.

3.4 The Building Regulations

The Building Regulations 2000 were issued under the Building Act 1984 and apply to England and Wales. The Regulations themselves are supported by Approved Documents that provide guidance on meeting the requirements of the Building Regulations. It is not mandatory to comply with the guidance given in the Approved Documents. Other methods of construction or design may be equally acceptable, providing they meet the Building Regulation requirements.

The Building Regulations that currently relate to access are:

Part M – Access to and Use of buildings
Part B – Fire Safety
Part K – Protection from Falling, Collision and Impact.

See 3.4.3, 4.1, 15.2.2, 15.13

3.4.1 Part M – Access to and use of buildings

Part M of the Building Regulations relates to access to and use of buildings. It applies to new buildings and some extensions, material alterations and changes of use.

See 3.4.2, 4.1

3.4.2 The Approved Document to Part M

This Approved Document offers guidance on Part M and identifies ways of meeting a number of objectives. It also considers design considerations and offers examples of technical solutions. However, the details shown represent only one way of addressing the requirements of the Regulation and other solutions matching the appropriate standard can always be considered.

Approved Document M requires reasonable provision to be made:

- for disabled people to be able to reach the principal entrance to the building, and certain other entrances, from the edge of the site or from on-site car parking areas
- so that elements of the building do not constitute a hazard for a person with a sight impairment
- so that people, including disabled people, can have access into and within, any storey of the building and to the facilities in the building
- for suitable accommodation for people in wheelchairs, or people with other impairments, in audience or spectator seating
- for sanitary accommodation for the users of the building, including disabled people.

The Approved Document also identifies the need for an "Access Statement". The form and scope of the statement will vary according to the size, nature and complexity of the building or environment being developed or altered. However, it should cover relevant issues, which may include:

- reasons for departing from the guidance, and the rationale for the adopted design where a designer wishes to depart from the guidance offered in the Approved Document to Part M
- the sources of advice and technical guidance adopted, including any consultation which is planned or which has been undertaken
- what the justification is if full access is not achieved in works to an existing building, particularly one of historic interest
- areas where access is restricted or not required.

See 3.4, 3.4.3, 4.1

3.4.3 Part B – Fire Safety

Part B of the Building Regulations applies to new build, refurbishment, extensions and alterations and sets out the requirements for fire safety. The Approved Document to Part B (AP B) gives guidance on meeting the requirements and makes reference to BS 5588: 1988, which gives detailed information on the design, construction and use of buildings. In AP B, only one reference is made to the appropriate means of escape for disabled people. It states:

"It may not be necessary to incorporate special structural measures to aid means of escape for the disabled. Management arrangements to provide assisted escape may be all that is necessary."

See 3.9, 15.2.2, 15.2.3, 15.8, 15.13

3.4.4 Part K– Protection from Falling, Collision and Impact

Part K covers the control of stairways, ramps and guards, and requires measures to be taken to reduce the risk of collision with open windows, skylights and ventilators projecting into circulation routes. It also covers measures designed to reduce the risk of injury when using various types of sliding or powered doors and gates.

In general, stairways, ramps and ladders which form part of the building must be designed, constructed and installed so the people may move safely between levels, in or about the building. This part of the Regulation (K1) applies to all areas of a building which need to be accessed, including those used for maintenance. Regulation K4, which requires steps to be taken to ensure that people moving in or around a building are protected from colliding with open windows, skylights or ventilators, does not apply to projections:

- which are at least 2 m above ground or floor level
- which project less than 100 mm into spaces.

Solutions offered by the Approved Document to K4 to reduce the risk of collision include the marking of projections with barriers or rails and the use of tactile surfaces to guide people away from the projection. These could have serious implications for disabled people if carried out inappropriately.

Door and safety features are covered in K5. This requires the opening and closing of doors and gates not to present a safety hazard to users. Details of vision panels and safety features for the use of sliding and/or power operated doors and gates are covered in this part of the Regulation.

3.5 Occupiers Liability Acts 1957 and 1984

Under the Occupiers Liability Act 1957 (OLA 57), the occupier of a building or area, owes a "common duty of care" to all visitors. That duty is to take such care "as in all the circumstances of the case is reasonable to see that the visitor will be reasonably safe in using the premises for which he or she is invited or permitted to be there".

Under the Occupiers Liability Act 1984 (OLA 84), an occupier may also owe a duty of care to "persons other than his visitors" often referred to as non-visitors. This may include trespassers.

For both Acts, what constitutes reasonable care will vary depending upon circumstances. The duty owed "in all the circumstances of the case" to disabled visitors, even if they are non-visitors under the OLA 84, may be different from that owed to non-disabled people, especially if a difference in the level of ability could have been foreseen.

3.6 Planning

The current planning system, which is based on legislation, orders and regulations, operates around a framework of three pieces of legislation:

1. The Town and Country Planning Act 1990
2. Planning (Listed Buildings and Conservation Areas) Act 1990
3. Planning and Compensation Act 1991.

Planning authorities are required to provide development plans which must be continually updated so that they remain relevant to all planning applications. When preparing such development plans, local authorities must take into account national and regional planning guidance relevant at the time. This guidance is identified in a number of Planning Policy Guidance notes (PPGs) and in Regional Planning Guidance notes (RPGs). The PPGs currently relevant to accessibility are:

- PPG1 General Policies and Principles
- PPG3 Housing
- PPG6 Town Centres and Retail Developments
- PPG12 Development Plans
- PPG13 Transport
- PPG15 Planning and the Historic Environment
- PPG17 Planning for Open Space, Sport and Recreation
- PPG25 Flooding.

In 2003, the Office of the Deputy Prime Minister (ODPM) issued a good practice guide entitled "Planning and Access for Disabled People". It addresses the need for the planning system to improve and enforce inclusive design principles when considering applications for planning consent. It also encourages local authorities to employ access officers to oversee access issues throughout the planning process and to provide expertise on access issues and solutions.

The guide also recommends that planning applicants are encouraged to submit an Access Statement to demonstrate their commitment to addressing access issues at the earliest opportunity. The statement should be seen as being complementary to that offered for approvals under Part M of the Building Regulations described earlier, rather than as a separate document. An access statement submitted at the planning stage could include statements which:

- demonstrate a commitment to achieving accessibility
- describe the strategic policies and approaches which will be adopted in achieving accessibility, including reference to the involvement of disabled people in the process
- demonstrate how management practices will maintain the strategic objectives of inclusion and accessibility
- identifies issues that will be addressed through ongoing management programmes such as, for example, planned maintenance.

See 4.6.2, 6.1, 9.4.7

3.7 BS 8300: 2001

Design of buildings and their approaches to meet the needs of disabled people – Code of Practice

BS 8300 offers detailed guidance on good practice in the design of domestic and non-domestic environments. The Code draws on research into the access needs of disabled people. This research considered issues such as limitations in reach, spatial requirements, and how the abilities of disabled people could be maximised when using the built environment.

BS 8300, which represents an amalgamation and updating of BS 5619: 1978 and BS 5810: 1979, considers a wide range of needs and contains sections covering building elements as well as particular building types. Detailed recommendations are given on car parking, setting down points and garaging, access routes to and around buildings, entering a building; horizontal circulation, vertical circulation, surfaces and communication aids, facilities in buildings, assembly areas, individual rooms and building types.

While BS 8300 is a guidance document rather than a statutory requirement, it is likely that the guidance given will be taken into account in considering what may be classed as reasonable provision under the DDA.

See 3.1, 4.1, 8.6.2, 8.6.3, 9.2.2, 11.3.2, 11.4, 11.7, 12.2.4, 12.4.2, 12.6.1, 13.1.5, 16.3.3, 16.11.4

3.8 BS 5588: 1988

Fire Precautions in the Design, Construction and Use of Buildings

The British Standard Code of Practice for means of escape is BS 5588. It covers different types and elements of buildings in all premises other than dwellings. BS 5588 Part 8 emphasises the role of management practices in escape arrangements for disabled people and introduces the concept of refuges (see also Chapter 15).

See 3.4.3, 3.9, 15.1.2, 15.2.2, 15.4

3.9 BS 9999

Code of Practice for Fire Safety in the Design, Construction and Use of Buildings

A proposed new standard to replace BS 5588 was undergoing public consultation at the end of 2003. BS 9999 has been developed to offer the most practical, relevant and up to date guidance to assist designers and managers of buildings in providing and managing reasonable means of escape for all building users.

The proposed code will cover fire safety management, means of escape, structural protection of escape facilities, the structural stability of a building in a fire, the provision of access, and facilities for fire fighting. The varying physical abilities and needs of occupants are considered in the code. Assessing how fire develops and the establishment of risk profiles are also included.

3.10 Human Rights Act 1998

The Human Rights Act 1998 came fully into force in October 2000. It incorporates into UK law, rights and freedoms guaranteed by the European Convention on Human Rights. Some of these rights may have significant implications for disabled people such as the right to education, right to life, respect for private and family life, and protection from inhuman and degrading treatment.

3.11 The Equal Treatment Directive 1975 (Amended 2002)

The Employers' Directive 2000 covers employment and vocational training. It prohibits discrimination on the grounds of sexual orientation, religion, disability, and age. It is intended that to amend the DDA to comply with this directive regulations will come into force in October 2004. It is proposed that these regulations will include the removal of the exemption for small employers (currently exempt from Part II of the DDA if they have fewer than 15 employees) and bring many of the occupations currently excluded from the provisions of the DDA within its remit.

4 Management

Management is a key issue in providing and maintaining the accessibility of services and employment opportunities in existing buildings. A well designed building or environment can be made difficult or impossible to use if management and maintenance practices do not consider access issues. Equally, the impact of inaccessible design in existing buildings may well be lessened to an acceptable, or reasonable, level if proper management policies are adopted and practised.

Table 4a The Inclusion Loop

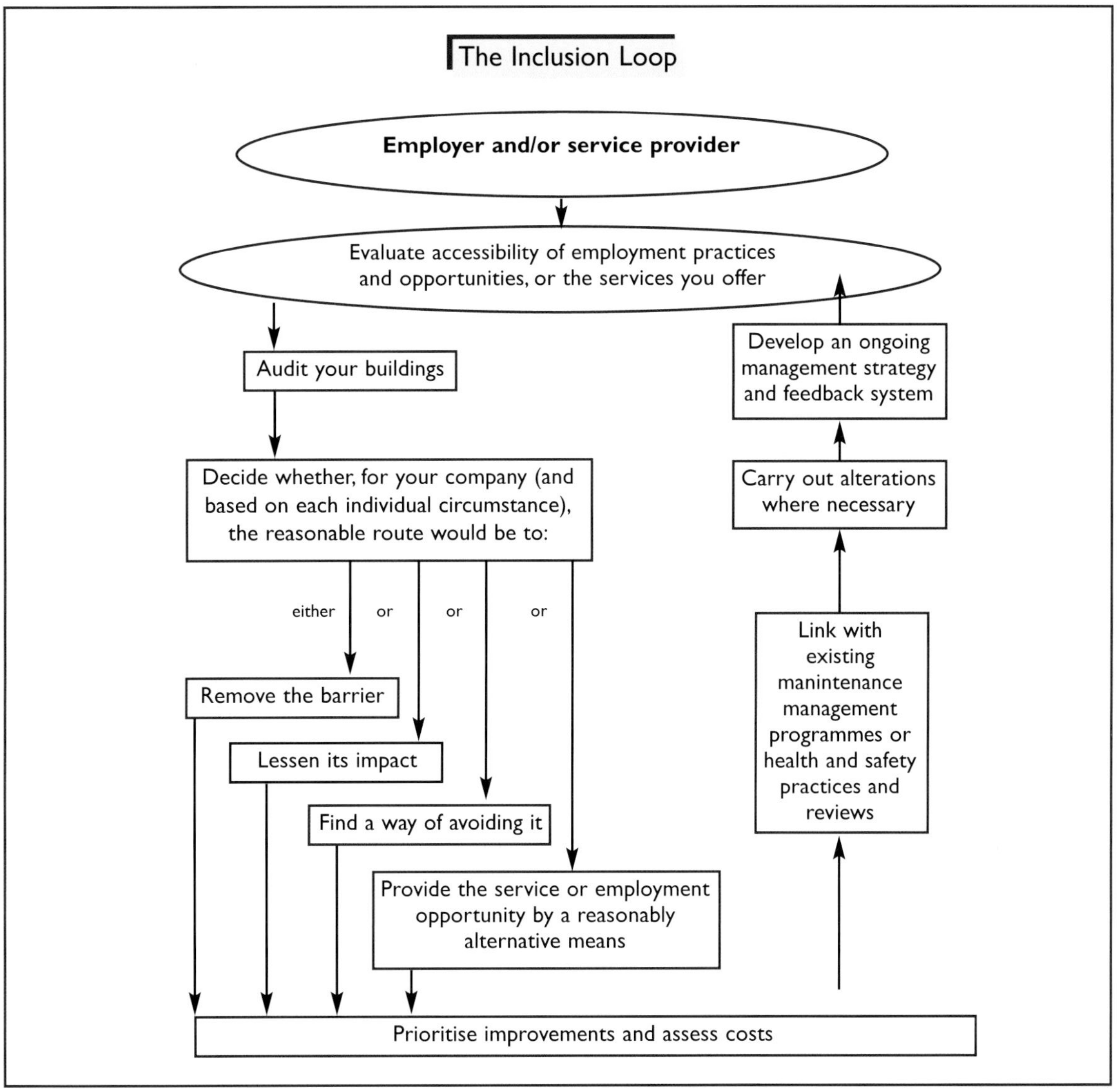

See 3.1, 3.8, 3.9, 4.5, 4.7.3, 4.7.6, 5.3.7, 6.6.3, 8.2.4, 8.3.4, 11.2.3, 14.2.3, 15.1.1, 15.4, 16.10.2, 16.11.3

Table 4a, identifies a procedure which could be incorporated into a management programme. The procedure would initially address issues related to the accessibility of an organisation's employment practices or services, and provide a process for ensuring their ongoing effectiveness.

4.1 Existing buildings

No reliable figures are available on the accessibility of the existing stock of public access buildings. Following the introduction of the Disability Discrimination Act 1995 (DDA), service providers and employers must consider accessibility and ensure that opportunities are available for both disabled and non-disabled people on an equal, non-discriminatory basis. Clearly, the number of buildings now required to have their accessibility assessed is considerable.

The Building Regulations can be used to ensure provision of a minimum standard of accessibility, and new guidance, such as BS 8300: 2001, offers examples of good practice, some of which go beyond the requirements of the Building Regulations. The revised Part M of the Building Regulations, and its supporting Approved Document, considerably increase the requirements related to accessibility and address more issues related to refurbishments and alterations than the previous Regulation. However, the new Part M still relates primarily to new build or substantial refurbishments. BS 8300 offers the best guidance for existing buildings but, although it may well be taken as an indication of reasonable provision under the DDA, not all the needs of disabled people in the population are included in the code.

4.1.1 Opportunities to make improvements

Elements of the built environment, such as buildings, transport infrastructure and pedestrian areas, often have a long life span, but that life is dynamic not static. There are many opportunities to make improvements throughout the life of a building. The skill is in understanding when activities occur that will allow those improvements to be carried out efficiently and cost effectively.

Within the general maintenance routine, there will be opportunities to replace any features which may be inaccessible or inappropriate, such as taps, toilet flushes, light fittings, poor decoration and poor floor finishes, when renewal takes place. Properly managed, many such improvements are related only to the selection of materials and equipment, and can often take place with little or no additional cost.

Opportunities may also occur in response to:

- redecoration programmes
- schedules of dilapidations
- changes in corporate identity (affecting, for example, company information and signage)
- work carried out to meet ongoing health and safety or environmental health legislation, such as redecorating, replacing controls, upgrading glass used in doors, upgrading lighting etc
- spaces that are allocated for new uses requiring new signage.

4.1.2 Landlord and tenant issues

In multi-tenanted buildings, where the landlord retains ownership of the common user parts, the landlord will be considered to be the service provider, for the purposes of the DDA. The service or services provided must actually be offered to members of the public or tenants occupying the building, rather than just existing for their benefit; it is a positive rather than an assumed service provision. Cleaning and lighting a shopping mall in a multi-tenanted retail development is an example of the provision of a service or services, provided by the landlord.

Common user parts include areas such as toilets, corridors, lifts, staircases and parking areas, all of which can be used by different tenants and people visiting the building. When considering the costs of making common user parts accessible, the landlord can recoup these costs from the existing tenants, only if it is specifically referred to in the service charge clause made with the tenant. If the service charge clause does not contain this proviso, the cost of any access work will be the responsibility of the landlord.

Existing tenants should therefore:

- clarify whether their service charge makes any provision for costs of access work
- consider the implications of carrying out any access improvements at the time of a rent review or lease renewal.

Access work could be considered to be an improvement under the terms of a lease. However, any improvements carried out by a tenant can be disregarded at the date of the next rent review or lease renewal because, under the terms of a lease, a hypothetical rather than an existing occupier should be taken into account. This could result in the scenario where an existing tenant may be penalised twice by:

1 Paying for the cost of the access work, for example, the installation of a lift.

2 Paying an increased rental at the time of renewal based on the original lettable floor area which has now been reduced by the introduction of a lift. (This is because, under the terms of the existing lease, the installation of the lift has been disregarded).

Leases all vary in their wording and content, and it is therefore vital that existing tenants obtain proper advice before carrying out access work in the premises that they occupy. It is also important for landlords to consult with existing tenants about any proposed improvements to common parts, because changes in management procedures may be sufficient in some multi-tenanted buildings.

4.1.3 Access guide

Service providers and employers should ensure their staff are aware of any shortcomings in the access to their service or employment opportunity, and do not give out, perhaps over the telephone, in handouts or in emails, information that could mislead a disabled person about the accessibility. This would be wrong in all situations but especially so in those areas where a disabled person may travel a long distance only to find a building or environment inaccessible.

If there are unavoidable barriers to physical access which it would not be reasonable to remove, making that information available to prospective users in an access guide will allow people to plan their visit, reserve parking places or just be aware of the areas where they may experience difficulties.

Information on accessible features is also useful in such a guide. If, for example, only one accessible toilet is provided, it would be useful for a disabled person to have information about whether it is a left or right hand transfer in case they are unable to use the facility.

Any guide developed must be readily available in alternate formats such as large print and audio tape.

4.1.4 Compromises

The use of many buildings will change with time and addressing the needs of all the users of the buildings must be a major objective. In certain situations where there are conflicts between, for example, historical importance, conservation, or physical constraints, it may mean that:

- compromise solutions may need to be accepted
- managed solutions, rather than alterations to the physical fabric, may be a better way of ensuring accessibility to the service or employment opportunity being offered.

However, what must never be compromised is the equality of access for both disabled and non-disabled people to the opportunities being offered. In the existing built environment, it may have to be acknowledged that an equal opportunity may not be the same as an identical opportunity.

See 5.2.2

4.2 Addressing inclusion

There are several tools available to assist in determining the accessibility of an existing building or environment, developing management strategies and planning future work. However, implementation of alterations and procedures will not benefit users or ensure legal obligations are met in the long-term if monitoring and feedback systems are not developed and maintained as part of an ongoing management policy.

4.3 Appraisal

Appraisal of a design is not a mechanical process. It must be undertaken with an understanding of the needs of the users, and especially disabled users, as well as understanding the technical and financial implications that may affect the appraisal of the proposed work. An appraisal should identify those areas where specialist knowledge is required. These may include:

- a very good understanding of the needs of disabled people, including the needs of any carers
- the ability to understand two dimensional plans and drawings
- knowledge of how the building or environment will be managed and used
- an understanding of the practicalities of construction and the approvals required
- knowledge of the various fittings and technologies which may enable disabled people to maximise independent living
- an understanding of building costs and details of where to obtain expert guidance.

People involved with access issues in the built environment do not necessarily need a construction background. Health professionals, such as occupational therapists and rehabilitation workers, and people with other expertise such as personal experience of disability, often have considerable experience in understanding the needs of disabled people and instigating alterations. The main requirement needed is an ability to understand and act, rather than a particular qualification.

4.3.1 Access appraisal

"Access appraisal" is the term usually associated with reviewing design drawings or details to assess the accessibility of a proposed building or for alterations to an existing one. It will usually be carried out by reviewing drawings and specifications, and involve consultations with the architect or designer. Difficulties can arise if the plans being considered are small scale or have been prepared before all the physical features of the site, such as levels, are known. To be effective, an access appraisal must be ongoing throughout the design and construction stages.

Some funding agencies, such as lottery funds, arts councils, trusts and charities, have their own access standards and insist on an access appraisal being carried out before considering applications for funding.

4.3.2 Access audits

An "access audit" is usually undertaken to establish how well an existing building or environment is performing in terms of accessibility and meeting the needs of its existing and potential users. An audit usually comprises:

- a site inspection
- an assessment of the use and management of the environment
- the preparation of a report identifying any problems, recommending improvements, prioritising the work and, in most cases, providing some indication of the costs involved.

Audits may be carried out to assess service provision or as part of a workplace assessment to identify the needs of a disabled employee and help identify changes that may be required.

See 4.3.4, 14.2.1

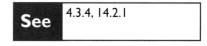

4.3.3 Staff training

Well-trained staff can make a positive contribution to the way in which disabled people use a building. Staff who are unaware of the needs of disabled people will often not respond appropriately, perhaps by shouting at someone who has difficulty hearing, refusing to assist or guide a person with a visual impairment, or giving written instructions to someone who is unable to read.

Staff also need to be trained in the use of equipment such as platform and stair lifts, induction loops etc. Training is also needed in management practices and procedures to ensure that they are appropriately delivered. This is especially important with respect to emergency escape procedures.

Staff training programmes must be structured, comprehensive, ongoing, and take into account any restrictions imposed by Health and Safety legislation.

See 6.3.6, 8.5.5, 10.4.4, 11.2.3

4.3.4 National Register of Access Consultants

The National Register is an independent resource for designers, building owners and managers seeking advice on how to make improvements in physical features or management practices, to meet obligations under the DDA and related legislation.

There are two types of membership:

- Auditors: experts in user needs and in identifying access problems and giving general advice on solutions
- Consultants: professionals who are experts in user needs and who are able to demonstrate a good understanding of construction related issues, gained either through working experience, a construction qualification or equivalent.

All members must undergo a professional interview and agree to operate in accordance with the Register's code of practice. Details are available on www.nrac.org.uk

4.4 Adding value

Improving access is increasingly seen as adding value to a building. Prospective buyers and new tenants are now more conscious of the need to consider accessibility as a basic requirement when comparing available property. The DDA, in ensuring that the needs of disabled people are addressed in the provision of services and employment opportunities, means that buildings and environments that are currently inaccessible are likely to be a liability, which will be reflected in capital and rental values.

4.5 Improving management practices and policies

The fundamental questions that need to be addressed when considering improvements for accessibility and implementation strategies are:

1. What work needs to be done?
2. When is the best time to do it?
3. Can the money be found?

Consideration should also be given to the consequences of sanctions resulting from postponing or not carrying out the work. Clearly, this will vary with respect to each individual case. What is common to all, however, is that taking no action is both unacceptable and potentially damaging to any service provider or employer.

4.5.1 Implementation by stages

It is important to plan for a satisfactory conclusion to any improvement works, even if it has to be achieved in stages. If funds are limited, it may be tempting to prioritise those jobs where a complaint has been made. However, if a full assessment and more comprehensive proposal identifies areas that would maximise accessibility, usability and cost effectiveness, then it is important to follow that route, as long as any obvious need for flexibility is not ignored.

4.6 Prioritising

4.6.1 Basic priorities

Whenever there is an opportunity to carry out improvements as part of a single refurbishment operation or planned maintenance programme, it should be taken. In these situations it is necessary to consider a fundamental priority of:

- getting into the building or environment
- providing equality of access to the goods, facilities, services and/or employment opportunities being offered

- appropriate use of facilities such as toilets, refreshment areas etc
- ensuring appropriate egress in an emergency.

4.6.2 Priorities based on use

The appropriate priority for improvements will vary from building to building and may be determined by, for example, the needs of a particular employee or group of employees, or the need to provide a service on a non-discriminating basis. Factors related to business planning may also affect priorities. It may be appropriate to examine how a building is actually used and, if there are restrictions on accessibility in one particular building that cannot be overcome, alternative solutions should be considered. An example would be changing the way business is conducted so that the service or employment can be offered in another building. If changes are appropriate, they must be changed for all customers and/or employees alike and not simply offer an alternative for disabled people only.

Planning is the key to:

- understanding the appropriate interventions required in various parts of the building or environment
- being ready to implement changes at the most appropriate time, in terms of user need and cost to the organisation
- determining if a permanent or temporary solution is necessary
- avoiding rework and its associated cost
- maintaining or improving the value of the company's assets
- improving the services offered to current and potential clients and maximising the opportunity to engage appropriate staff
- identifying "quick wins", changes or improvements that can have maximum impact with minimum cost and disruption.

Priorities and programmes should be developed through consultation with management, users, and organisations representing users and employees. It is essential that both non-disabled and disabled people are appropriately represented in each of these groups.

See 4.3.2

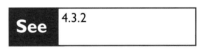

4.7 Strategies

4.7.1 Forming a strategy

A strategy should be formed around a planned programme of implementation as well as identifying those issues that will have maximum effect in the shortest possible time or with the most cost benefit. It is important not to let the best be the enemy of the good. What is needed is effective accessibility, and this is not necessarily the most expensive solution.

Disabled people will enjoy using a building or an environment that is transparent in its accessibility and does not appear as though it has simply been adapted to meet their needs. Good information that allows disabled people to plan their journey and to be advised of any obstacles they may encounter, will encourage them to make that journey and participate in the service or employment opportunity on offer. This may well affect demand by increasing the numbers of both disabled and non-disabled people who wish to use a service.

4.7.2 Consultation

In an existing building, it may not be possible to follow design guidance to the letter. Consultation will ensure that all parties concerned have an opportunity to suggest the work required, together with any alternatives and compromises.

Clients, users, user groups and designers, should all be involved in managing the building or developing a brief for identifying the objectives of the work and how they can be achieved, both in terms of procedural and physical changes. Proper consultation at an early stage will also allow issues which sometimes present conflicting requirements, such as security, accessibility, fire evacuation etc, to be discussed. Any conflicts can then be addressed, drawing on as wide a range of views and experience as possible.

4.7.3 Cost benefit analysis

The most expensive improvements will not necessarily be those which result in the greatest benefit. What is needed is a coordinated approach, based on a true understanding of what is needed, and when. By introducing practices that will address any shortcomings in the accessibility of a building and identifying the appropriate time to undertake improvements, management procedures can assist in reducing rework, and the associated waste of valuable resources.

For example, if a lift which is due for replacement in four or five years time is not totally accessible, a management procedure could be introduced to remove or lessen the impact of the obstacle. With careful planning, perhaps by providing assistance to all users of the lift, the lift may well be usable for the remainder of its full life and the cost of replacing it now can be offset against other, more immediate accessibility issues. However, this type of decision must be taken on the merits of an individual circumstance. There is no "one size fits all" solution here.

4.7.4 An access plan

For an existing building, consideration should be given to developing an "access plan", which is a strategy for improving accessibility originating from an access audit. An access plan can assist an organisation in identifying opportunities for change and be a useful tool for meeting obligations imposed by the DDA and other related access legislation. Following the initial audit to establish the physical and non-physical barriers for disabled people, an access plan should be developed which identifies a plan of action for:

- implementing the findings
- introducing procedures for the ongoing updating of the audits
- training staff in user needs awareness and disability issues
- informing disabled people of improvements carried out
- regularly reviewing the effectiveness of adjustments made, and what positive action is needed to maintain the improvements
- developing and updating schedules of work to be carried out, including costs
- linking audit findings to maintenance management programmes.

4.7.5 Publicity

If improvements have been carried out and a good level of accessibility has been achieved in an existing building, it is essential to publicise this information. Local access groups, newspapers and journals, radio coverage and a web page, are all good vehicles for disseminating information.

See 4.8, 4.9.1

4.7.6 Linking accessibility to maintenance management

The adoption of good management practices, such as planned maintenance programmes, can offer major opportunities in:

- improving accessibility
- ensuring accessibility becomes a key part of the management strategy of the building or environment
- reducing the risk of lost opportunities.

The access audit can identify maintenance issues that affect accessibility, and planned maintenance programmes can be used to ensure that there is a continuing commitment to maintain access, with funding available to repair and replace accessibility features when required.

Once accessibility has been improved, perhaps by the installation of good lighting or a platform lift, a commitment is made which was not previously present. The installation needs to be regularly inspected by appropriately qualified people and priorities must be established. Money must also be available, perhaps at short notice, for repair or replacement.

If a facility is not working when it is required by a disabled person, it may be construed as being discriminatory against those people who need to use that facility to access a service or employment opportunity. It could be argued that the management procedure covering the inspection, testing and maintenance of the facility is, in itself, discriminatory.

Improving accessibility using colour and luminance contrast can be undertaken during any redecoration work. Selecting different colours does not cost more money, but it must be planned for in terms of what to use, and where to use it.

Good provision is essential – effective on-going management is critical.

See 4.1.1, 8.4.4, 11.2.2

4.8 Implementation by strategies

This section offers owners and managers of environments a strategy that can be used to develop an ongoing evaluation of management and implementation activities.

The brief

- **What are the policy objectives?**
  Usually several policies operate in combination, eg to increase the use (numbers of customers), to make it possible to employ disabled staff and, to upgrade the building with a view to increasing its rental or sale value.

- **What improvements are possible?**
  The access audit should provide this information.

- **What is the priority for specific improvements?**
  Review the possible improvements in the light of the policy objectives, bearing in mind that individual improvements may be ineffective (for example, providing a ramp to the entrance if the toilets are inaccessible). Identify a ranking system that suits the needs of particular clients or situations.

- **Are there conflicting issues to be addressed?**
  These might include means of escape, security, energy conservation, cost management, staffing, different user needs, conservation of historic buildings. Existing contractual arrangements with service companies, such as cleaning, security etc, may also conflict with proposed changes in management procedures. How will such issues be resolved?

- **Who should be involved?**
  Identify responsibilities, allocate duties, assess need to appoint consultants, define channels of communication and the consultation procedures.

The budget

- **What is a realistic budget to achieve each level of priority?**
  In some cases, the budget may come from separate sources and/or appear under different headings (for example, maintenance, replacement of equipment, upgrading for a new use, specific improvements to access for disabled people).

- **Is there the political will to support the budget?**
  The question has to be asked. If there is any doubt, a positive strategy will be needed to emphasise the benefits of improvement and the legal implications of failing to carry them out.

- **What money is available?**
  Known sums available now and at future dates.

- **Are there any potential sources of funding?**
  This might be from charitable funds and sources available for special building types to whom applications could be made (for example, money from Lottery funding). Employers may be able to obtain money to adapt the workplace for new and existing disabled members of staff (for example, "Access to Work").

- **Will more money become available at a later stage?**
  What needs to be done to secure it?

- **Who has responsibility for the cost of improvements?**
  Are they aware of the costs?

- **Will equipment supplied for improvements be subject to VAT?**
  At the time of writing, supplies may be zero rated when made to a charity (but not to a local authority). Such things as ramps, stairlifts, induction loops and signs can be zero rated to charities.

- **Will costs be met from mainstream funding?**
  Will reliance have to be placed only on the maintenance budget?

- **Can the cost of improvements to accessibility be justified in terms of the company perspective?**
  This will have to be considered against the overall strategy for the company and may include consideration of the life of the building (physically and commercially), the operations of the company and its future plans, if any, for the building.

- **Is the cost such that it might be considered unreasonable under the DDA 1995?**
  This will depend on several factors, all of which are unique to the issue being considered. The size of the company, the disruption caused, what other work has been carried out, the plans for the future, and what management practices could be put in place that still offer "equality" in the provision of the service or employment opportunity, are some factors that will be considered if there is a challenge in the court or an industrial tribunal. What is appropriate to one company in one situation is unlikely to be applicable to another company, even when considering an identical access issue.
- **Can alterations benefit both disabled and non-disabled people?**
- **What specialist advice will be needed?**
  Are the fees covered?
- **Is there allowance for feedback from use?**
  An appraisal and consultation after completion of each stage may reveal a need for additional work.
- **Maintenance, insurance?**
  For lifts etc.

The programme

- **Does it make sense to make improvements in stages?**
  This may be to spread the cost or to align expenditure with other work.
- **How will the building function, for all users, whilst improvements are being made?**
- **What approvals are needed and how long will they take?**
  Assess approval requirements (eg planning, building regulations, listed buildings consent, fire officer, ground landlord) and include the time required in the programme.
- **Are other improvements, alterations, extensions planned?**
  Is there a conflict? Could work be programmed to benefit from economies of scale or temporary work such as scaffolding?
- **How is the other building work organised?**
  For example, is it feasible to extend existing consultancies or contracts?
- **What is the most suitable time to carry out improvements?**
  For example, between terms or exhibitions, in winter or summer.
- **Can the building work be restricted to zones so that the rest of the building can function normally and reduce the need for extra cleaning?**
- **How will the public find out that the building has been improved?**
  For example, is there an information strategy that will include publicity locally (newspapers, radio), nationally (web page) or in accessibility statements about the building? When is publicity to be arranged, and by whom?

See 9.2.6, 15.1.1

4.9 Feedback and post-occupancy evaluation

Feedback is an important element of improving accessibility. It allows for the essential fine-tuning that ensures improvements have met their objectives. It also allows for any difficulties identified to be addressed, so they are not repeated.

Completing the information loop (see Table 4a) requires positive management action to identify how the improvements are being used. Lack of feedback often means that clients, designers, legislators and disabled people themselves, will not be aware of how their ideas work in practice.

See 4.8.1, 4.9.2

4.9.1 Post-occupancy evaluation

A post-occupancy evaluation draws together information about how the building is being used and can be a useful tool in establishing:

- how effective the improvements have been
- if more disabled people are now using a building or service
- whether management are making the most effective use of the improvements
- whether there has been sufficient publicity to make people aware that improvements have been made.

The evaluation can be carried out using interviews or focus groups, suggestion boxes and questionnaires, and might include an audit of the building or environment after the improvements have been completed.

4.9.2 Feedback

Once gathered, feedback must be used effectively. This can be done by:

- arranging to hold design reviews and making accessibility a main item on the agenda
- making the information gathered available to the whole design team
- collecting and indexing examples of good practice which are readily available.

5 Communication, wayfinding and information

5.1 The need for good information for everyone

For many disabled people, access to information is just as important as access to the environment itself. However, all users need good information if their use of an environment is to be effective. The principles that apply to good provision of information to disabled people is equally relevant to meet the needs of non-disabled users.

Most users of environments will gather information using the five senses of sight, hearing, touch, smell and taste. Approximately 70–75 per cent of information is received visually and about 10–15 per cent audibly, and information can be provided visually, audibly or with the use of tactile features and surfaces. Additional "clues" about environments are sometimes provided by aromas, for example in supermarkets, cafés, etc.

In most cases, the common method of providing information is by the visual sign. It is known that 82 per cent of the visually impaired population have the use of some residual vision which, if maximised by the provision of clear information, can greatly increase their independence and safety. Without maximising the visual information available, or providing it in alternative ways, such as audibly or with tactile features, there is clearly an information deficit which hinders wayfinding and orientation.

People who are deaf or hard of hearing may avoid asking for information in case they are unable to understand the answer, so they rely heavily on signage to give them the information they need.

It is essential that all users, and disabled people in particular, are able to receive information and to process it rapidly so that they are able to complete a journey or identify a feature as easily as possible.

5.1.1 Misinformation

Providing poor or misleading information can have serious consequences and should always be avoided. For example, giving a person who relies on tactile surfaces the wrong information is potentially far more dangerous than giving no information at all.

A lack of information will usually mean that a person remains alert and wary; incorrect information can lead to a false sense of security. Areas where this type of information is of paramount importance would be, for example, on platforms in transport environments, at the top and bottom of stairs and at dropped kerbs.

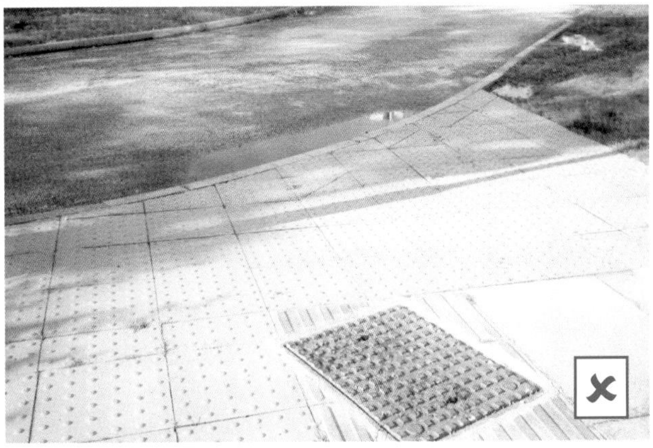

1. An example of the very poor use of tactile surfaces as an information provider. Someone trying to gain information from this tactile surface, would need to interpret very confusing messages. The blister pavement is the wrong colour for an uncontrolled crossing, the long sections of the surface used to give directional information (bottom right) are lost in a heavily embossed manhole cover.

5.2 Sources of information

5.2.1 Consistent detailing

The approach to providing information should be based on consistent detailing throughout a building or an environment. Disabled people should not be required to face a new challenge each time they unlock a door or operate a door opener. Accessible routes should be logical in their design.

Features needed to assist movement or to give information, such as handrails, lift controls, light switches, the location of accessible toilets in relation to standard toilet accommodation, and the location of stairs relative to lifts, should not present further challenges every time they are required. Consistent detailing should aim to ensure that all users can easily familiarise themselves with the layout and operation of the building.

5.2.2 Access guides

In some buildings it may not be possible to remove a physical barrier or, because of the nature of the business, to adopt policies and practices that allow independent access to the service or the employment opportunity. Such constraints might occur because of, for example, an inability to obtain Listed Building Consent for alterations, or because of restrictions in the security arrangements.

If there are unavoidable barriers to access, and this must be judged on the merits of each individual example or case, publishing that information so that a disabled person can effectively plan his or her journey, should be considered. An access guide can be sent out in advance to allow people to plan their visit, reserve parking places, take an accompanying person or just be aware that restrictions on their independent access are present.

See 4.1.3

5.2.3 Information on services available

Information on the services available for getting to a building or environment could be provided. This could include the location of railway or bus stations, bus stops, drop off points (for private cars or taxis), and the approximate distances to be travelled to reach the accessible entrance. Surface finishes of paths such as loose gravel, cobbles etc, which are likely to cause difficulty for the disabled, could also be identified. If services are provided to offer users some form of assisted travel, such as customer transport, then this should be made available. Long, detailed descriptions are not necessary, but information highlighting potential hazards, even if they are outside the control of the service provider, will assist users when planning their journey.

5.2.4 Clarity of instructions

The presence and operation of services, such as lifts, stairlifts, platform lifts, induction loops, text telephones and visual and audible alarm systems, must be made clear to users. Information and instructions must be available in a format appropriate to the needs of the user.

5.2.5 Location and design

Instructions for the presence and operation of services should be appropriately displayed in terms of viewing distance, height, legibility and tactility (where appropriate). Some signs and detailed instructions may have to be duplicated at different heights or in different positions to allow for convenient close vision, especially in areas that may be congested, such as those close to lifts or stairs.

5.2.6 The use of sign language

Sign language, which uses both visual expressions and hand gestures, is used by some deaf or hard of hearing people as a structured method of communication. It has its own vocabulary, grammar and syntax and is used all over the world, although its makeup does vary between countries. In Britain, British Sign Language (BSL) is mainly used although, as with any language, there can be regional variations in the words used and in the meanings of words. For some deaf people, BSL is their first language and they may not use written or spoken English at all.

For this reason, some BSL users will be able to lip read if the environmental conditions, such as colour and lighting, are appropriate, and the lip movements of the person they are communicating with are clear. However, some BSL users will not be able to communicate by lip reading. The precise number of BSL users is not known but the Royal National Institute for Deaf People (RNID) has estimated that there are between 30 000 and 70 000 BSL users in the UK.

See 2.2, 10.4.4

5.3 Signage

5.3.1 Clear information

Legible and easily understandable directions, information and instructions should be provided to clearly identify:

- accessible routes
- the characteristics of a route which may not be fully accessible and which may present navigating difficulties for some disabled people.

Clear signs should be provided as part of a comprehensive signing scheme. Signs should be conspicuous and provide useful information. At a base level, a sign should say to the person who needs to use it "I am the sign you need to make a decision, read me". The information given should also take into account that the reader of the sign may not speak the language of the sign and will therefore, place great importance on pictograms or icons. This will be especially important in transport environments or areas with multi-cultural populations.

The techniques to be adopted in providing signs that are useful, meaningful and conspicuous include:

- holistic approach – provide a signage system not just individual signs
- language – be consistent in terminology and plain English
- symbols – use recognised pictograms wherever possible
- positioning – show important signs in obvious, consistent and logical positions (see picture 2)
- lighting – ensure that signs are well illuminated
- text/pictogram size – use an appropriate size relative to viewing distance
- text/pictogram style – use a simple san serif font and standard symbols
- tactility – ensure that information that can be touched is tactile
- colour and contrast – ensure adequate contrast of information with sign and sign with supporting wall
- surface finish – use a non-reflective finish for all elements.

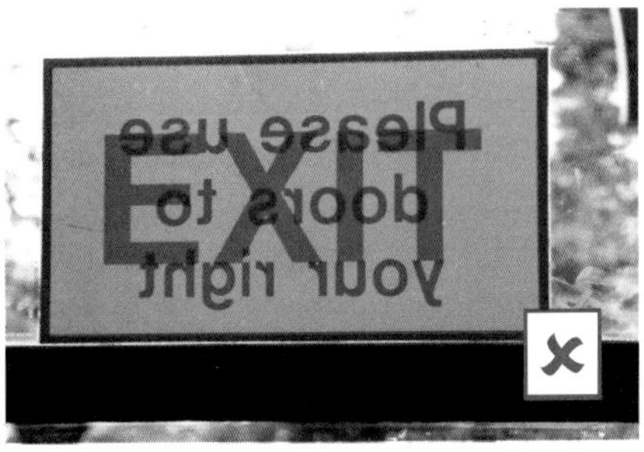

2. When signs are positioned care must be taken to ensure that, unlike here, they will actually work in use

See 5.1.1

5.3.2 Signs in existing buildings

Good signage is particularly important in existing buildings that may have been extended or developed over the years and which may have lessened any logic to the original layout. For example, alternative entrances, alternative access routes, lifts or facilities in non-logical positions, may have been provided and will need to be signed appropriately.

Signs in buildings may also have accumulated over the years with older, redundant signage not being removed. Refurbishment and active, on-going, management practices that review existing signage, are good opportunities to rationalise what exists with what is required (see also Chapter 4).

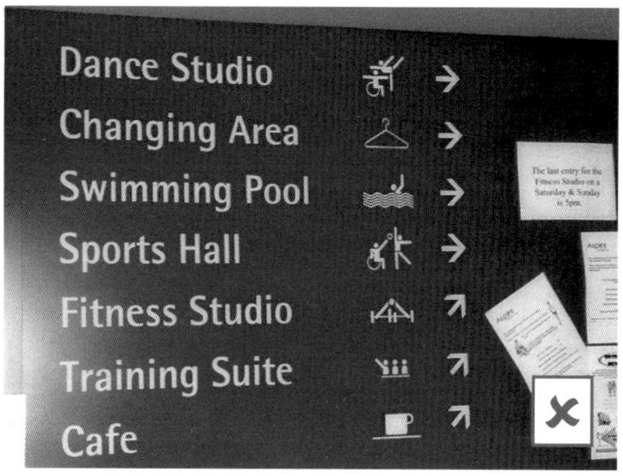

3. Good use of font and pictograms but the sign is made very confusing by the unmanaged use of temporary signage.

5.3.3 Information on available facilities

On arrival at a building, everyone should be able to determine what facilities are available. Facilities that are of particular benefit to disabled people should be clearly identified. Information should also be available in alternative formats such as large print and audio format. In general, there will be a lesser need to provide Braille of all documents, but procedures should be in place to provide information in Braille if it is the only format the disabled person can use. Induction loops to assist hearing aid users to gain information, should always be provided at reception desks, information desks, ticket booths and other critical areas, for example, at counters where pharmaceuticals are being dispensed. (see also Chapter 9 and section 5.7).

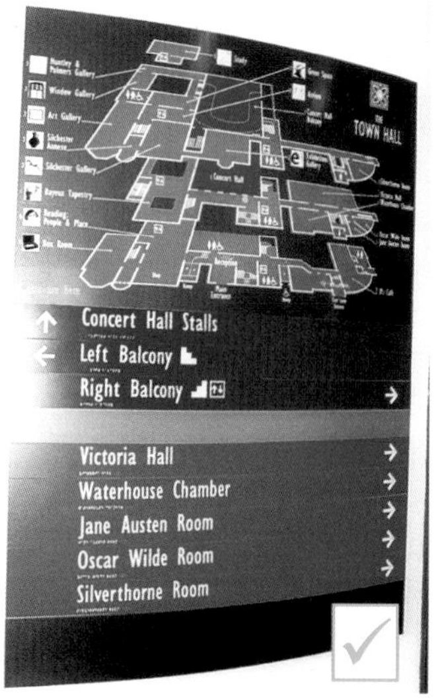

4. Good information sign with good use of colour contrast, pictograms, directional information and Braille. However, placing the directional arrows closer to the text would have improved clarity.

5.3.4 Text or pictogram size

Text and pictograms should be large enough to be seen clearly at normal viewing distance. A rule of thumb is a minimum of 100 mm and a maximum of 170 mm at a viewing distance of 3 m. This can be adjusted pro rata for longer or shorter distances, but there must be a minimum character size of 20 mm for signs that will be read at close range. The *Sign Design Guide* published by the Sign Design Society offers full guidance in this area.

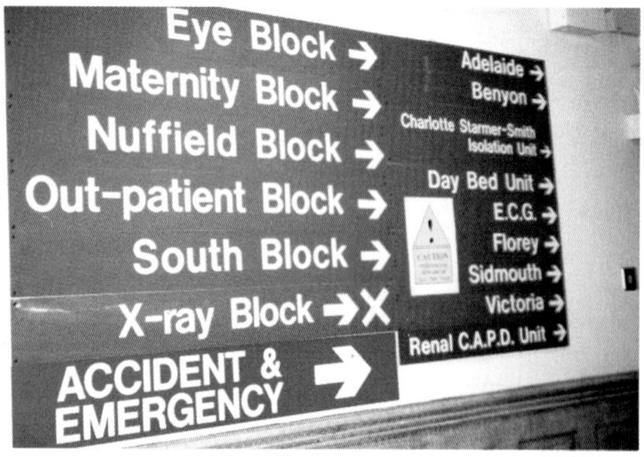

6. Symbols are good practice and the use of an "**X**" as a symbol to denote "**X-ray**" seems logical – but what does "**X-ray block →X**" mean. Does it mean "go this way" or "don't go this way"?
It meant something to the designer, but what does it mean to the users?

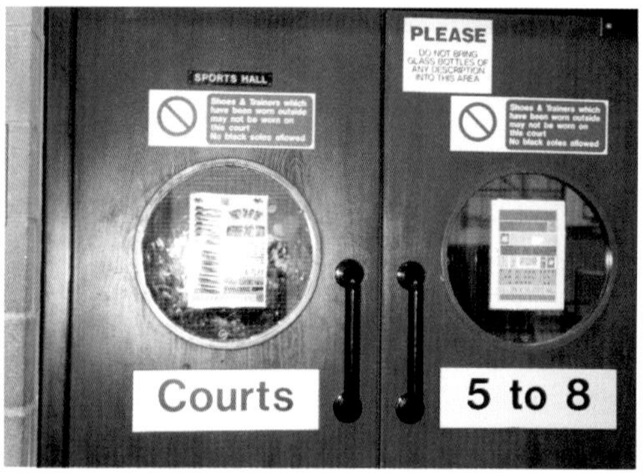

5. Always avoid information overload

See 5.3.1, 5.3.6, 5.7

5.3.5 Tactility on signage

Tactility should be introduced to signage by embossing, never engraving, the letters or symbols. This is very important for signs that can be read by touch. Signs that can be touched might also include Braille. Good practice for tactile signs suggests that:

- the depth of embossing should be a minimum 1 mm with the edges chamfered or slightly rounded
- lettering or symbols should have a minimum height of 15 mm and a maximum height of 25 mm
- signs that incorporate upper case lettering only should not be used. Capitals and lower case lettering should be used to assist the reading of the word by pattern recognition (a method which can be very important for people who experience dyslexia, learning disabilities, restricted vision or whose first language is not the one used on the sign)
- Braille can be helpful on signs but its use, in terms of the amount of information given in Braille on a sign, should be limited. Braille signs are more easily read if they are on an inclined surface, rather than in the vertical plane. Grade 1 Braille should be used and, as the specification for Braille dimensions is strictly controlled, there is no room for deviation.

See 5.4

5.3.6 Colour and contrast on signage

The ease with which a sign can be read will, to a large extent, depend on the effectiveness of the colour and contrast used. In general:

- a signboard should be well contrasted with the wall on which it will be mounted or, if freestanding or hanging, the background against which it will be viewed
- the text or pictogram should contrast with the board
- signage should be unobstructed and visible at all times.

Borders to sign boards can accentuate the contrast of the sign with its background, but care should always be taken to ensure that the relationship between the contrast of the lettering with the signboard and the signboard with the background, is appropriate. For example, black lettering on a white signboard would offer maximum contrast, but if the sign was then fixed to a white wall, it would not be sufficiently distinguishable. In that situation, it would be preferable to have white lettering on a black signboard. What is important is not only to look at the contrast on the sign, but how it will appear in use.

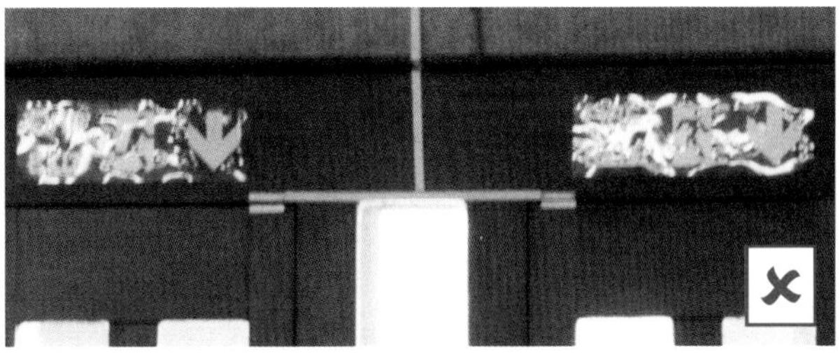

7. Poor choice of surface finish makes these important emergency signs unreadable. This could have been prevented at no extra cost, if the issues had been understood.

See 6.3.5, 8.6.5

5.3.7 Temporary signage

Temporary signage can be very confusing and its use should be controlled by active management procedures. Out of date signage, signs that are in inappropriate formats or printed on reflective surfaces or covered with reflective materials, must be avoided. If signs are important and needed long term, they should be appropriately provided in a permanent format. If they are not important or long term, they should be removed.

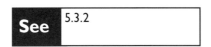

See 5.3.2

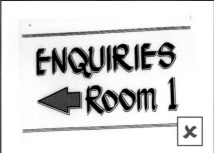

8. A busy font, upper case lettering and a light background on a light wall make temporary signs like this one difficult for many disabled people to use.
Good management practices should monitor the use of temporary signage.

5.4 Information gained through touch

The sense of touch can be used to gain many pieces of information, the most obvious of which are variations in temperature, surface finish, shape and moisture content. Buildings that are designed to maximise the sense of touch, can be a considerable information source, but careful thought is needed in understanding not only what tactile clues to use, but also where they should be used. On a circulation route, changes in floor finish are important sources of information, and helpful in locating features and positions. In this respect, people with visual impairments are often comfortable using floor surfaces that provide sufficient resistance and grip, whereas floors that suddenly deflect or are slippery can make many people, and especially those with a visual impairment, feel uneasy and less confident.

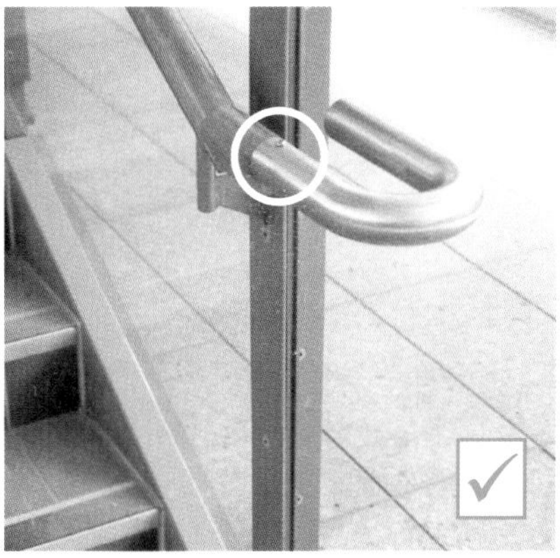

9. A tactile feature can offer valuable assistance to people gaining information through touch.

Accompanied by careful use of colour contrast, changes in floor surface can give a tactile clue to denote, for example, the swing area or direction of swing of doors, routes to reception desks or the presence of a lift, and can give warning of imminent changes in floor level. In some cases, a simple change between a hard and soft floor finish, can provide sufficient tactile and aural information to distinguish, for example, a circulation route from other areas.

Hands can be used to gain tactile information but, unlike the feet, they are not in constant contact with the environment being used. Here, a better understanding of where information is likely to be found is more critical. Information could be given using, for example, tactile letters on door handles (perhaps giving visually impaired people an indication of the direction of exits to be used in an emergency). Raised studs on handrails can give an indication of the floor level reached, or embossed arrows could indicate the direction of exits. Tactile signals such as these are simple and inexpensive to install, but they can considerably improve the amount of information available and the usability of the building for some users. Tactile surfaces should always be used consistently and in accordance with the latest guidance.

5.5 Colour and lighting

Colours can be used to identify routes within a building or to assist people in determining particular zones within a building. Lighting can also be used to highlight the presence of features such as lifts, without the need for a written sign. In the use of colour and lighting as an information source, there are great opportunities for creativity, but care must be taken. Chapter 13 covers design and use issues in greater detail.

5.6 Induction loops and infrared systems

5.6.1 Induction loops

An induction loop system incorporates a microphone and an amplifier/transmitter, with the output connected to a continuous loop of wire that encircles a given space and acts as an aerial. Induction loop systems should conform to BS 7594: 1993 and BS EN 60118-4.

When in operation, the system is used by a number of hearing aid users simultaneously. Induction loops should be tested to determine the optimum frequency to suit all users. Magnetic interference from, for example electrical equipment, can seriously affect the performance of an induction loop. Induction loops should never be used if there is a risk of "spill over" of the loop signal to an adjoining area, something that may compromise confidentiality.

See 2.2, 5.2.4, 5.3.3, 5.6.2, 10.4.3

5.6.2 Infrared systems

In areas where confidentiality or containment of transmitted sound is required, or where local inference is likely to prevent an induction loop system being used, an infrared system should be considered. Such systems are also of benefit if more than one channel is required for audio description or translations on a second channel. Infrared amplification systems use an infrared diode linked to a microphone to send signals to a light sensitive receiver usually incorporated into headphones. The managers of an event or building usually supply the headphones to individuals attending particular events. They are commonly found in theatres and concert halls.

Advantages of infrared systems are that they:

- offer a higher quality of sound reception than the induction loop
- avoid spill over of sound into adjacent spaces
- can be provided with neck loops, which are mini-induction loops, for people wishing to use their personal hearing aids
- can be used by people without a hearing impairment who may simply wish to listen to the sound without interference from the background noise of the audience around them.

Infrared systems do commit the service provider or the employer to on-going management resources which are not required by the installation of an induction loop. For example, retrieval of infrared receivers that have been loaned to users for performances, maintenance, hygiene and security of the system, all need to be accounted for, and there is a need for on-going training of staff in the use of the system.

5.6.3 Inductive couplers

To assist people who wear a hearing aid that has an inductive pick-up, an inductive coupler and additional volume control should be fitted in all public or visitor telephones, entry phones and emergency telephones in lifts.

5.6.4 Signs and instructions

Standard signs showing that an induction loop, infrared system or induction coupler is available, should always be provided. Suitable instructions on how to use these systems should also be provided in alterative formats.

5.6.5 Visible reinforcement

A user who is deaf or hard of hearing will not be able to hear an audible sound such as a distant bell or buzzer. Therefore, visible confirmation is also needed. The use of audible systems that do not have a visible backup must be avoided. Public address systems should always be supplemented by flashing lights, illuminated signs or visual display boards, to reinforce the spoken message.

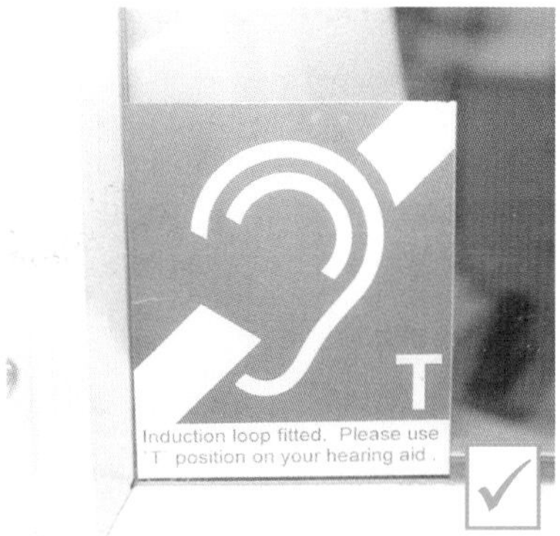

10. Clear symbol showing the presence of an induction loop.

5.7 Other forms of information

For some information, text is not the only or the best way to communicate. Where people need to locate a route through a complex site or building, a plan or model may be more helpful than the use of the written word or a symbol. However, if tactile maps are used, expert advice must be taken to ensure they are both accurate and readable.

Other forms of communication can include audio-taped information or messages delivered to the user using radio or infrared transmissions.

5.8 Audible communication

Information given audibly should always be available in printed format and visually.

5.8.1 Audible signs

The use of audible signs can be advantageous in some environments. Signs may produce continuous or intermittent sounds, spoken messages at regular intervals, and be activated by proximity devices, pressure buttons or push switches. Common audible systems are those used in lifts, on travellators and at controlled pedestrian crossings.

5.9 Communications in an emergency

Alarm/alerting systems such as flashing beacons and vibrating devices that work in conjunction with conventional emergency alarm systems, should be installed to assist those users who are deaf or hard of hearing. Care must be taken if consideration is being given to the installation of flashing/stroboscopic light systems as they may induce confusion, disorientation and, in some people, epileptic seizures.

See also Chapter 15 for information on the use of powered emergency wayfinding systems.

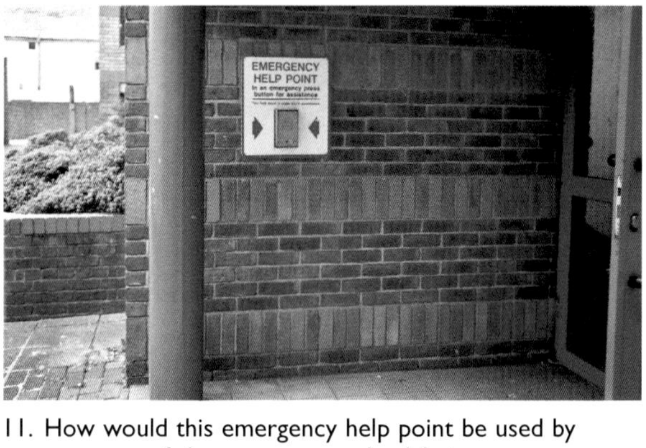

11. How would this emergency help point be used by someone of short stature, a wheelchair user or a person who is deaf or hard of hearing?

6 Historic buildings

6.1 Introduction

It is important that historic buildings are conserved for future generations because they are a finite resource with cultural significance. For the purposes of this chapter, the definition of historic buildings has been taken from Part M 2003, paragraph 0.17. This states that historic buildings include:

1 Listed buildings.

2 Buildings situated in conservation areas.

3 Buildings which are of architectural and historical interest and which are referred to as a material consideration in a local authority's development plan.

4 Buildings of architectural and historic interest within national parks, areas of outstanding natural beauty, and world heritage sites.

5 Vernacular buildings of traditional form and construction.

There are currently 371 591 Listed Buildings and 19 446 Scheduled Monuments (Heritage Counts, 2003). Historic buildings are protected by two pieces of legislation:

- the Planning, Listed Buildings and Conservation Areas Act 1990
- the Ancient Monuments and Archaeological Areas Act 1979.

Under the current legislation, it is necessary to obtain Listed Building Consent (LBC) from the relevant local planning authority for any proposed works of demolition, alteration or extension, which affect the existing character of a listed building, including any object or structure within its curtilage (English Heritage, 2003). If a detailed proposal is refused LBC, it may still be possible to achieve an alternative and acceptable design solution.

LBC is also required for any internal and external alterations to a property, irrespective of whether these are identified separately in the list description. These alterations can include changes to entrances, door widening, lift installation, provision of ramps and handrails etc. LBC may also be necessary for any temporary alterations, which may be required in advance of any permanent alterations to an existing building. However, temporary solutions are not a substitute for long-term solutions and it should be recognised that some temporary solutions are more temporary than others.

The Disability Discrimination Act 1995 does not override existing planning legislation or the need for LBC. Also, some ecclesiastical buildings are exempt from LBC provided they are from "exempt denominations" that have their own approval system. Ecclesiastical exemptions do not override the service provisions of the DDA. In all cases, the provision for inclusive access to historic buildings needs to be looked at as part of an integrated process reflecting a flexible and pragmatic approach wherever possible, but accepting that compromises may have to be made to protect the architectural or historic importance of the existing building. There may be some situations where designing for inclusive access will be acceptable only if these compromises can be made. The aim should always be for dignified access to and within an historic building. When considering inclusive design in an existing historic building, an access audit and an Access Appraisal should be carried out at the earliest opportunity. A strategy including an access plan should also be considered.

One of the difficult issues when considering inclusive access for existing historic buildings will be reconciling the different pieces of legislation, ie Building Regulations, the Approved Document to Part M, the DDA and Listed Building Consent. It is only as Case Law becomes more widely established that the question of what constitutes a reasonable adjustment will become clearer and easier to clarify. However, it is important to recognise that access issues in an existing historic building are more likely to be resolved amicably, if there is thorough and ongoing consultation with all relevant parties including the access officer, the planning department, local access groups, funding institutions, English Heritage and Cadw (Welsh Historic Monuments). In some situations, it may be advisable to discuss the proposed plans for the building with the relevant building control officer before submission. This could avoid lengthy time delays in the planning process.

See 4.3.1, 4.3.2, 4.7.4, 8.7.5, 9.2.4, 9.3.5

6.2 Alterations to historic buildings

When considering alterations to an historic building, it is important to establish what is important or significant about the building. This is a vital first step in thinking about changes. Buildings can be significant in many different ways. The layout may be particularly important, or the building may have important historical associations or there may be important remains below ground. The better the understanding of what is important, the easier it will be to design appropriate new work.

Information about the significance of a building may be obtained from a conservation plan or statement, where these exist, or from a meeting with the conservation officer from the relevant local authority.

The process of reconciling the importance of the building and its environment with the needs of its users is a significant part of the access planning process. This should be a logical, well-documented and coherent process from access audit to access plan to Listed Building Consent to access statement for approval under Part M of the Building Regulations. The access statement is a way of reconciling the demands in the Approved Document Part M where generic solutions may be impractical when applied to existing buildings. BS 7913: 1998 *The Principles of the Conservation of Historic Buildings* gives guidance on achieving balances between different interests in decisions affecting historic buildings.

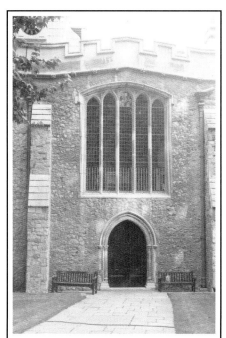

1. Alterations to the fabric of the building may not be possible – but can the external approach be landscaped to remove the obstacle of an entrance step?

The management of design issues (see Chapter 4) also plays a key role in providing for inclusive access in existing historic buildings. If a building is managed efficiently and sympathetically, this will minimise the need for physical intervention. There may also be opportunities for improving access as part of other future work, for example, when funding has been allocated for restoration work. It is important to recognise that specifying work to make an existing historic building accessible, is not just a one-off exercise, but needs to be viewed as part of an ongoing process taking advantage of other opportunities in future work programmes.

The most relevant guidance for carrying out alterations and improving access to historic properties is contained in the publication from English Heritage *Easy Access to Historic Properties* 1995. This guidance, which is due to be updated in 2004, currently focuses on the needs of people with mobility impairments and there is minimal information about providing facilities for people with sensory impairments. It is intended for owners and occupiers of historic buildings who have particular responsibilities as service providers under the DDA, as well as professional people such as architects, planners and access consultants. However, the guidelines do not cover policies, practices and procedures, or the general design issues, referred to in the DDA. The proposed guidelines will focus mainly on the needs of wheelchair users and people with limited mobility, because carrying out alterations for physical access requirements will place the greatest demand upon the existing fabric of the building.

It is important that any proposed improvements or alterations that are carried out on a historic building should:

- have regard to the existing structure by enhancing rather than detracting from the design and appearance
- be carried out sympathetically
- wherever possible, use building materials that are similar to or have and affinity with the original
- have regard to whether the proposed changes are reversible and could be removed with minimum damage at a future date
- recognise that every part of a listed building is protected, both the outside and the inside of the existing structure
- ensure that any plans for proposed work are drawn up after consultation with bodies who are sensitive to both conservation and access issues.

There are good examples where alterations have incorporated traditional building materials that blend with and match the existing structure and the original design is not dramatically affected. Removal or alteration of a significant feature within a historic building should be avoided. It is advisable to consult the relevant local authority conservation officer as early as possible when considering alterations to a historic property, because the time taken to obtain the necessary permissions and consents is often longer than those required for unlisted buildings.

Currently, no direct funding is available from either English Heritage or the Heritage Lottery Fund for specific access improvements to existing historic buildings. However, funding may be available from the Heritage Lottery Fund if the proposed alterations form part of a larger project. (English Heritage, 2003).

6.3 Design issues

It is difficult to apply standard design guidance to historic buildings because of their individual character and appearance. Each property will present its own unique access problems and there will be different recommendations, solutions and management issues, depending upon the existing architectural features.

See 6.1, 6.3.3, 6.3.5, 8.7.5, 9.2.4, 9.3.5

6.3.1 Approach and entrance

The pedestrian approach to existing historic buildings can often incorporate materials such as gravel, stone slabs and loose cobbles. These surfaces can be difficult in terms of access, particularly for wheelchair users and people with mobility impairments (see also Chapters 8, 9, 10, 11 and 12).

It is essential to ensure that all surfaces are well maintained and that, when any uneven surfaces are re-laid, the historic nature of the footpath is not significantly altered (see Chapter 7 – Case study of St Mary's Church, Kintbury).

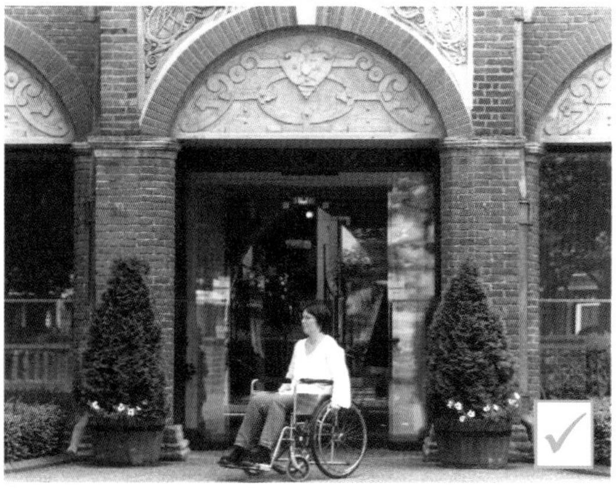

2. A good example of an accessible entrance into an historic building.

The entrance into an historic building is often one of the most impressive features of that building. When considering inclusive access, it is important that any changes do not compromise the original design. One way of achieving this is by the use of similar materials and detailing which will blend in with the original construction. For example, if a ramp and handrails are required, it is not necessary for the handrails to contrast so strongly with the background to make them stand out more prominently than any other feature in that building. The only requirement is that the handrail should be easily identified for inclusive access into the building.

See 8.11–8.1.4, 8.2.1, 8.2.2, 9.1.1–9.1.5, 9.2.1–9.2.6, 9.6.1–9.6.7

6.3.2 Horizontal circulation

When carrying out work on an historic building, it is important that damage is either avoided or kept to an absolute minimum. For doors that are particularly heavy to open, the use of automatic door-opening mechanisms or the introduction of a bell to call assistance can be used to improve accessibility. Where existing door ironmongery cannot be replaced by lever handles owing to its architectural or historic significance, alternative solutions may have to be considered such as providing additional staff to assist with door opening, or fitting an automatic door opening mechanism. However, for any door alterations in an existing building, it is essential that any damage to existing doorframes and finishes is minimised. Care should also be taken to ensure that features such as panelling, dado rails, skirting boards and historic floor surfaces, particularly if they are fragile and valuable, are protected. This may result in the use of temporary or removable guardrails or temporary coverings. Temporary structures, because they can be removed easily, may not require any special permission, but they should not interfere with the special character of the building. If there is any doubt whether or not consent is needed for temporary alterations, the local authority's conservation officer should be consulted.

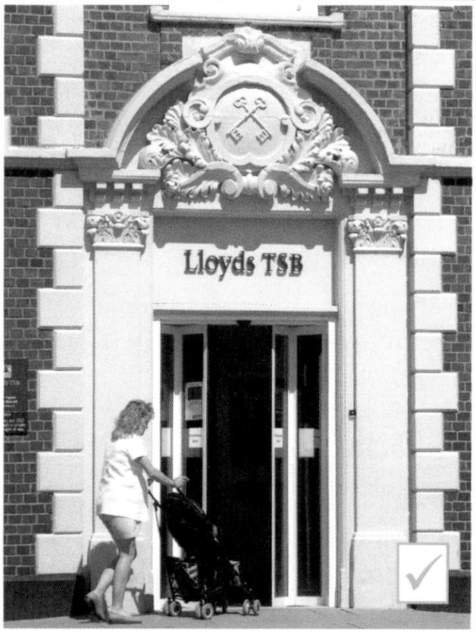

3. Another good example of an accessible entrance into an historic building.

Existing historic buildings are often characterised by narrow doors and uneven floors and the removal of such features is unlikely to constitute a reasonable adjustment under the DDA. Alterations to management procedures or changes in service provision are more likely to be appropriate in these cases, such as providing an alternative route through the building to avoid the feature, or relocating a service to another, more accessible part of the building. Compromises should also be considered subject to consultation.

See 3.2.5, 11.1.1

6.3.3 Vertical circulation

Staircases

The main staircase in an existing historic building is usually one of the most important features in terms of its architectural and historic significance. It can be difficult to carry out any significant alterations, and alternatives may have to be considered such as the use of any other secondary staircases which are less architecturally important.

If there is only one existing staircase, subtle alterations may have to be considered such as:

- the use of additional lighting to improve the illumination of each step
- nosings to highlight the edge of each step or stair
- alterations to the existing handrail design
- the use of carpeting to improve the contrast for visually impaired people as an alternative to the provision of tactile warning surfaces.

Handrails

Tactile features can be used to identify handrails, as an alternative to using colour and contrast. However, if any new handrails are recommended for an historic building, it is imperative that the necessary drawings showing the proposed details are submitted for consent as soon as possible, and enough time is allocated for alternative solutions if initial permissions are refused or require resubmission.

There is no guarantee that initial approvals will always be granted and often there will have to be a compromise to the original submission. The only advantage with handrails is that they can usually be removed with minimal damage to the building fabric, so they are relatively independent of the structure.

Ramps

If a ramp is required in an historic building and it is physically problematic to carry out this work, for example, owing to space restrictions or damage to the fabric of the building, consideration should be given to introducing a temporary or portable ramp as an alternative solution. However, it is essential that the necessary staff training and management procedures are in place, particularly if a wheelchair user needs to use a portable ramp, and that it does not provide a tripping hazard for other users of the building. Portable ramps are likely to have less visual impact on an existing building because, unlike temporary ramps, they can be removed and stored away when not in use.

The amount of existing appropriate storage space available within a building is a key consideration when using any portable items of equipment, particularly in an historic building. However, some access solutions, such as the provision of, for example, lifts, wider corridors and additional staircases, may place increasing demands on that building in terms of space. This highlights the fact that there are often direct consequences to carrying out improvements in an existing building.

Platform lifts (see also Chapters 12 and 15)

Short rise platform lifts are often less intrusive than a long ramp with handrails, and are more suitable for an existing historic building, where there is a change in level between one and four metres. However, it may be difficult to identify space for a platform lift within an existing historic building, so other alternative solutions should be considered such as installing a direct acting ram lift, which does not require a pit underneath the platform and is likely to have less impact on the building fabric. The disadvantage of this type of lift compared with a scissor action platform lift, is that the overhead guide rails are more obtrusive than the guarding required for a platform lift.

Passenger lifts (see also Chapters 12 and 15)

The introduction of a passenger lift is the best solution when considering inclusive access to the upper floors of a building. In a building that does not have any historic significance, a lift can be installed without too many problems, providing there is sufficient space for constructing a lift shaft of adequate size, and the necessary structural calculations have been carried out.

In historic buildings this may be more difficult to achieve and it may be necessary to consider installing the lift into:

- a new extension
- a less historically sensitive area of the building.

In most cases, building work for a lift is not reversible so alterations will be seen as being permanent. However, it is possible to install lifts in historic buildings and there are good examples where this has been successfully carried out. Also, the use of modern lift technology can reduce or avoid the need for overruns and lift pits.

Stairlifts (see also Chapters 12 and 15)

Installing a stairlift into an existing building can require less space and be significantly less of an intervention on the historic fabric than constructing a vertical lift shaft. Stairlifts fitted to the stair treads are usually the most practical solution for an historic building. This is because they are less intrusive than those that require fittings at skirting, lower wall or dado level, where the existing fabric, for example, panelling, may be irreversibly damaged.

6.3.4 Lighting

Different lighting schemes can be used as a method of identifying the edges of steps on a staircase in an historic building. This will assist all users but particularly those with a sensory impairment. However, care should be taken to ensure that the introduction of new lighting does not cause glare or confusing shadows. The introduction of window blinds should be considered as a method of eliminating glare at certain times of the day.

In some historic buildings, lower levels of lighting are necessary, for example, to display historic artefacts in a museum where a high level of lighting could damage the exhibits. In these cases, assistance should be given, for example, by providing seating so that people have a place to rest or pause and become accustomed to the lower levels of lighting, before continuing with the display. Other examples of assistance to compensate for lack of adequate lighting include the provision of handrails to give tactile information and the illumination of individual hazards such as an isolated step or projecting furniture (see also Chapter 13 Lighting).

See 5.5, 8.10.1, 9.4.6, 12.9, 13.1, 13.1.1, 13.1.2, 13.1.4, 13.1.6, 15.13, 15.13.1, 15.13.2

6.3.5 Communication

Signage, tactile surfaces, colour contrast and induction loops

The introduction of new signage or the modification of existing signage can present a major problem in an historic building. It is often difficult to find suitable places within a building for fixing signage without it changing the character or spoiling the existing appearance, for example in an impressive lobby or foyer. One solution may be to consider introducing freestanding signage that does not involve damage to the walls or ceilings of the existing structure. If freestanding signage is used care should be taken to ensure that all obvious routes through the building are not obstructed and that the signage does not cause a tripping hazard. If there is no alternative but to fix signage to the existing fabric, it will be necessary to consider the fixings used and their compatibility with the existing materials within the building.

The scope for using colour and contrast as a way of highlighting certain features within a building to assist wayfinding and navigation, is much more limited in an historic building. Alternative solutions may have to be considered, for example, the use of different tactile surfaces to assist in identifying important features within the building, such as stairs, lifts or handrails.

There is also limited scope for altering the acoustic environment within an existing historic building because it has often been furnished and decorated in a style which is in keeping with how that building was originally used and occupied in earlier centuries. For example, in some historic buildings, the layout of furniture within rooms has been designed to recreate the original ambience by the use of specially chosen soft furnishings, carpets and furniture. If the acoustic level is altered by, for example, changing the flooring or the curtains, this may completely change the character of that individual room or building.

The introduction of induction loops for people with a hearing impairment will not affect the structural fabric or architectural importance and therefore can be installed in any existing historic building.

6.3.6 Facilities

If it is impossible to identify space within a building of historic interest for accessible toilet facilities, it may be possible to provide them in within an adjacent accessible area. This may be a public area or one that is mainly intended for staff, but where management practices are in place to ensure members of the public could also use it. If it is the latter, it is important to consider security aspects and staff training procedures, particularly if people have to go into areas of the building that are not normally open to members of the public.

Information about unavoidable barriers to accessibility could be made available in an access guide. This will allow disabled people to plan their journey and visit effectively. See also Chapter 16.

See 3.4.2, 4.7.6, 5.2.2, 5.3.3, 8.4.1

7 Case studies

7.1 Four Winds, Pacific Quay, Glasgow

Introduction

The property is a Grade A listed building which was originally constructed in 1894 as a steam powered hydraulic pumping station. It supplied the cranes used for loading and unloading cargo from the ships docked on the Clyde.

The building was originally designed by the architects Burnet, Son and Campbell and is a mixture of Italian Gothic and Romanesque styles. It is currently used as the Glasgow offices of Buro Happold Engineers.

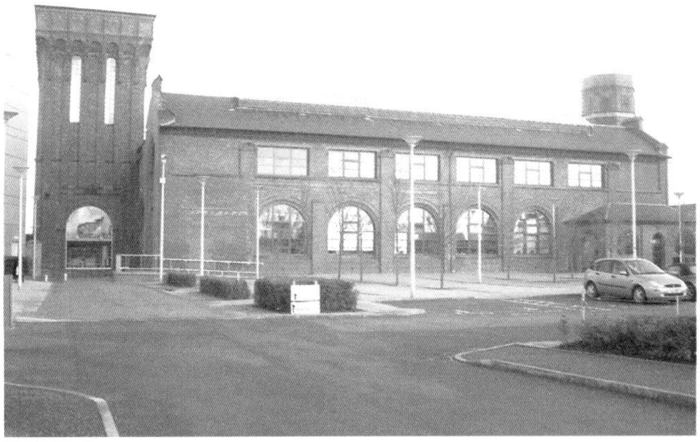

1 Accesible parking bays are located close to the building entrance.

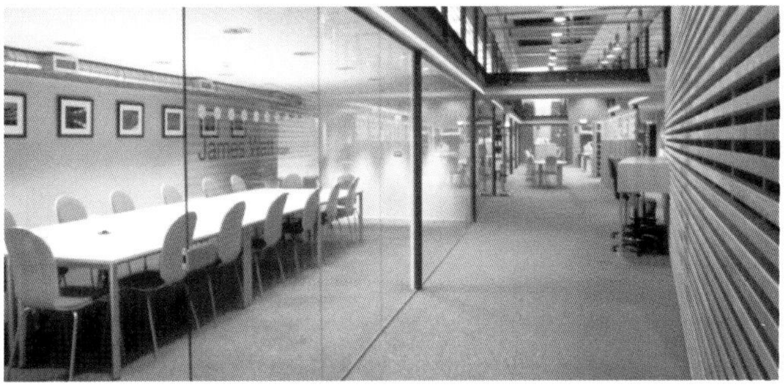

2 The finish on the wall helps to indicate the route through the space.

The improvements

Approach

Accessible parking bays are located near the entrance and dropped kerbs are provided. A new smooth accessible route has been laid which runs parallel with the existing cobbled route. Signage to the office was provided as part of the improvement works. Public transport links to the office are poor and inaccessible.

Entry

During the refurbishment of the building, a new entrance layout was designed which complements the listed nature of the property. Both stepped and ramped access is provided to the office, allowing independent access for all users.

A proximity card access control system, where an identity card just has to be presented 4–6 inches inches from the reader, to be was chosen over swipe card systems, because they have been more difficult for people with limited manual dexterity to use outside normal office hours. During office hours the reception staff controls the entry system.

Arrival

The reception desk is directly opposite the entrance and is easy to locate and identify. The area in front of the desk is unobstructed and the receptionist is framed by a single colour display that facilitates lip reading. The reception desk incorporates a choice of counter heights, which makes it easier for a wheelchair user to approach the desk closely. An induction loop has been installed.

Horizontal circulation

The design team had considerable freedom in the design and fit-out of the empty shell. Accessibility was considered early on in the project and has resulted in a successful and innovative inclusive office environment in which the accessible features are passive rather than prescriptive.

Short pile carpets allow wheelchair users to move easily throughout the space. Colour schemes and signage have been designed and installed to reflect good practice. Features within the scheme, such as the timber wall and the overhead light fittings, help to orientate a visitor and identify circulation routes.

Possible hazards such as the columns have been highlighted using colour and luminance contrast. Doorways are highlighted in a similar manner to make them distinctive from their surrounding walls. All doors have lever handles.

Even though the glazed screens of the main meeting rooms help to create an open feeling office space, they can be difficult to see for people with visual impairments.

The design of the manifestation (markings to make the presence of the glass more obvious), on the glass on the glass is less effective in practice than originally intended. The narrow doors to the meeting rooms are difficult to distinguish and should be more effectively highlighted.

Vertical circulation

The decision not to provide lift access to the mezzanine floor of the office was affected by a number of factors: these included the listed nature of the building, the size of the mezzanine floor space, and the management decision to duplicate all facilities on the ground floor.

While informal meeting spaces are distributed throughout the office, designated meeting rooms are located on the ground floor.

There are closed risers on all the stairs, and nosings have been highlighted with colour and luminance contrast. The timber handrails have an easy to grip profile. The handrails finish with a positive end.

Effective continuing management of the facilities has been essential to maintain the accessible nature of the office.

Services

All office furniture has been designed to provide an accessible working environment. The furniture contrasts in colour and luminance with the floor, and the lighting scheme has been designed to eliminate glare. There was a conscious design decision to maximise the use of natural light in the office, but electrically operated blinds have been installed to diffuse sunlight when necessary.

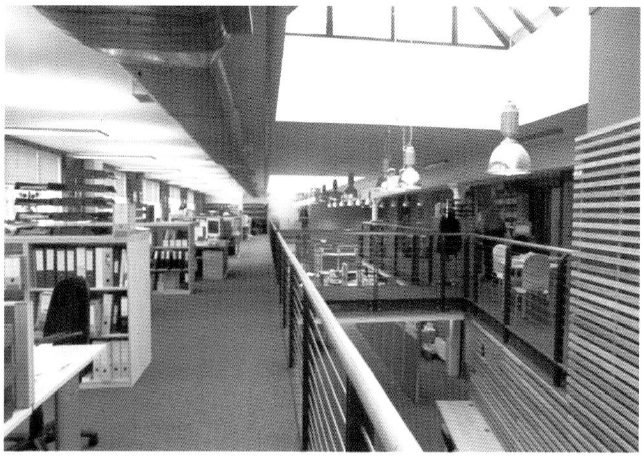

3 The circulation route is well defined. Handrails have a circular profile in accordance with best practice.

Printing services are duplicated on both levels of the office and have been grouped together and separated from the main working environment. This reduces any distraction caused by the noise produced by such equipment and the flow of people through these areas.

A text-phone is available to employees and an induction loop is provided at the front reception desk to aid communication in this busy area.

The fire alarm system generates both an audible signal for assisting people with a visual impairment and a flashing beacon to assist people with a hearing impairment.

Facilities

A unisex accessible toilet conforming to BS 8300: 2001 has been collocated with the standard toilet provision on the ground floor of the building. Originally the building had male, female and accessible toilet provision but because a high proportion of employees are male, a management decision was taken which resulted in the unisex accessible toilet also being used as the female toilet.

Refreshment areas are duplicated on both floors of the office.

The Tower improvements

In late November 2003, the refurbishment of the tower adjoining the main office space was completed. The move into this vacant space was seen as an opportunity to extend the office space and improve the functionality of the office.

The historic nature of the building, the limited increase in floor space on the upper levels, and the previous decision not to provide lift access to the mezzanine floor all influenced the design of the tower space.

The original management decision to locate unique services on the ground floor was applied to the tower works, leading to the judgment that a new café area, allowing workers a space to relax/hold informal meetings, should be situated downstairs, while the mezzanine level would become an extension of the general office space, and the gallery level a further informal meeting space.

Design features within the new tower area are consistent with all other areas of the office, the risers on all stairs are closed and nosings highlighted with colour and luminance contrast, while handrails are formed in wood, have an easy to grip profile and finish at a definite ending.

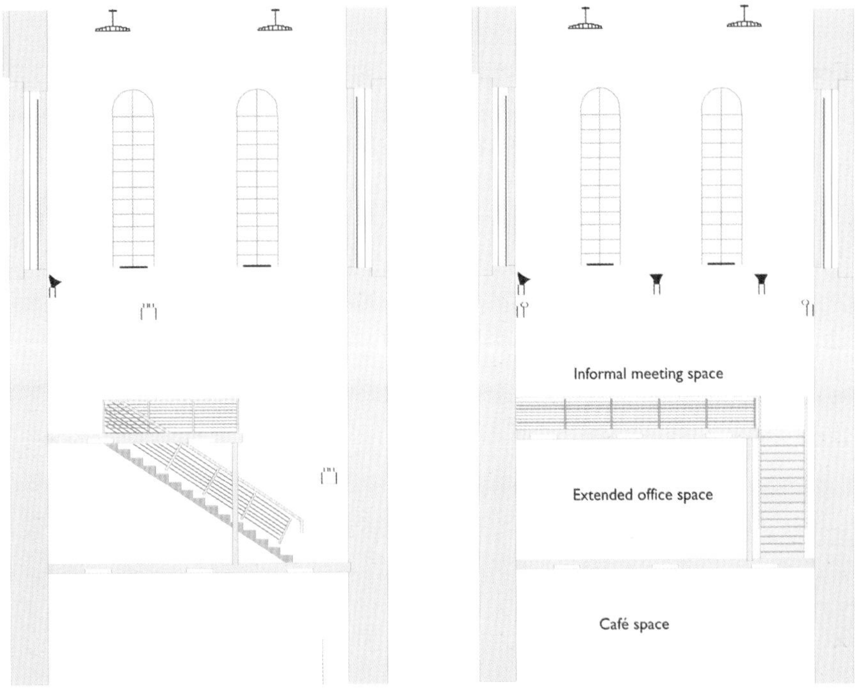

Figure 7a Section view of tower showing unique spaces located on ground floor only.

How the work was done

Designing an accessible office space within a listed building, while retaining its character, architectural integrity and place within the industrial heritage of Glasgow, would provide a considerable challenge to any design team.

However, by considering the needs of disabled people from the outset and working with the design company's own access team throughout the project, the project team has successfully created an environment which is aesthetically acceptable, enjoyable to work in, and accessible.

During the recent extension of the office into the tower, the design team and office management jointly considered the needs of disabled people and the impact of any new design on the existing access strategy within the office. This ensured an improved office that continues to emphasise the values of accessible design.

Lessons to learn

- By considering the needs of disabled users throughout the project, it is possible to provide an accessible building that benefits all users.
- Although an office, or any building, can be designed to be accessible, continuing management of the environment is essential to the building remaining so. This includes the day-to-day management of workspaces and meeting areas, as well as more fundamental design or layout issues.
- Prescriptive management decisions are often unnecessary if all staff carefully consider their actions and are aware of the specific needs of disabled people.
- It was important to provide a well-designed colour and tonal contrast scheme in areas of a building, and to increase accessibility passively and enhance the working environment for everyone.
- When improvements are made to a building, it is important to consider the impact these changes will have for disabled people. It is vital to have a complete understanding of the current and past management decisions concerning accessibility within the building, ensuring that refurbishments do not have a detrimental effect on the accessible nature of an office.
- Although the individual members of a design team working on a project may change, the ethos of the group should remain focused on the needs of all office users, including people with disabilities.
- The transport links and pedestrian routes to the site can have a big impact on how accessible the building is to disabled people. However, changes to this important aspect of accessibility are often not within the control of the design team.

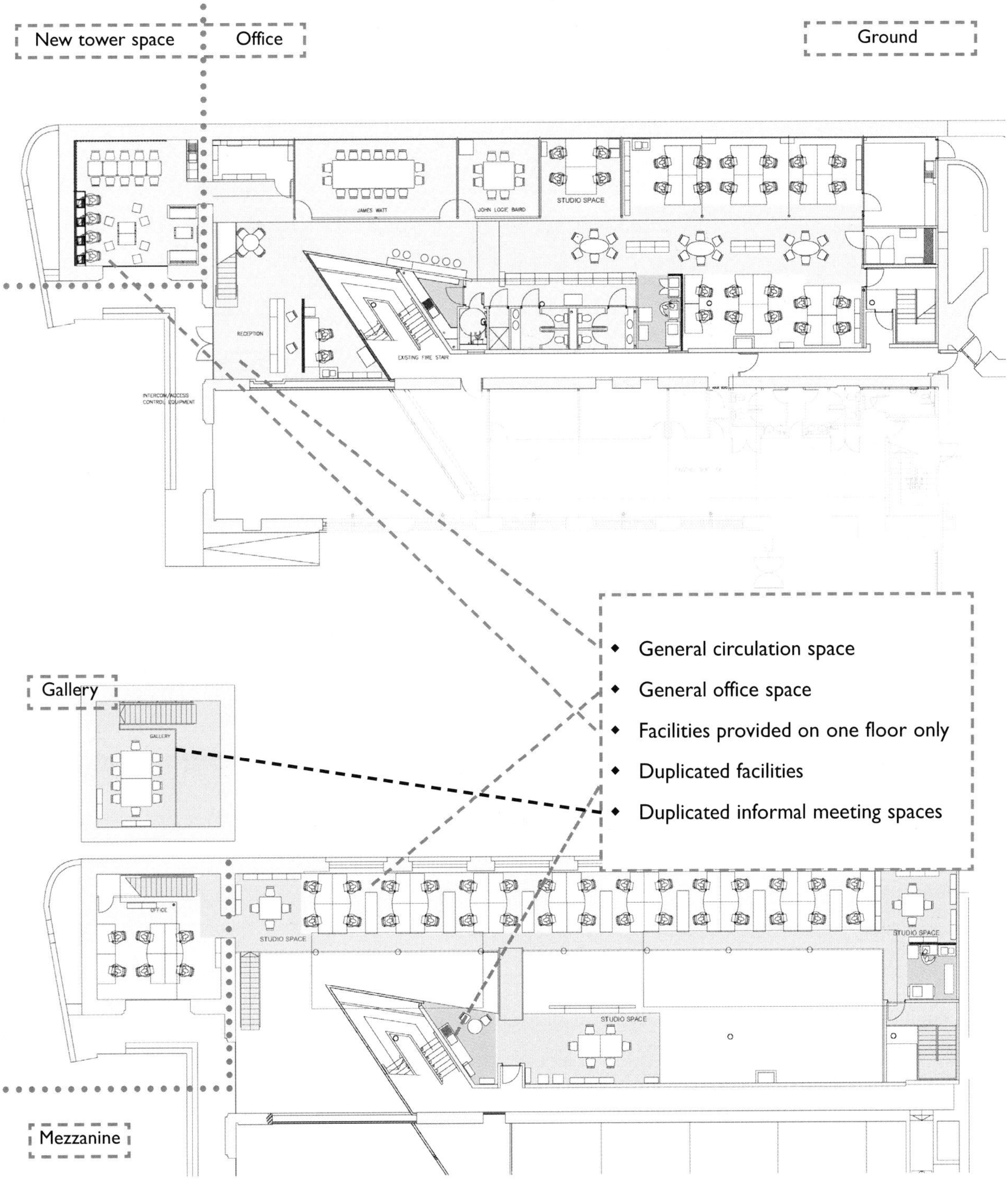

Figure 7b Plan view of Four Winds showing office space uses.

7.2 Manchester Piccadilly main line station

Introduction

Manchester Piccadilly station was originally designed by W Baker and L H Moorsom. The design, comprising a trussed arch roof 95 ft wide and 680 ft long, was completed in 1866. A further two comparable spans were added 15 years later.

The station was known as Manchester London Road until redevelopment works in the 1960s.

Piccadilly is one of three main stations in Manchester, and handles more than 55 000 passengers and 1000 trains every day. The station acts as a terminus for Intercity services, a through station for regional services and as a local metro link tram station.

A £20 million refurbishment process carried out between 1998 and 2000 introduced a replacement lighting system, an up-to-date signage strategy and new platform surfaces, while the decorative train shed brickwork was cleaned and the original roof replaced, which involved the renewal of more than 10 000 individual panes of glass.

A subsequent award-winning £60 million redevelopment phase has further transformed the station into a world-class travel facility.

The improvements

In line with the brief, a new, larger concourse (7000 m^2) spanning two levels was introduced. The lower platform level concourse provides 2000 m^2 of retail accommodation, a new travel centre, passenger facilities and toilets, whilst the upper level concourse includes a modern space with a pub and restaurants making use of the balcony seating overlooking the trains, public areas and the city of Manchester.

The new north block provides enlarged accommodation for numerous train operating companies and a management and control suite.

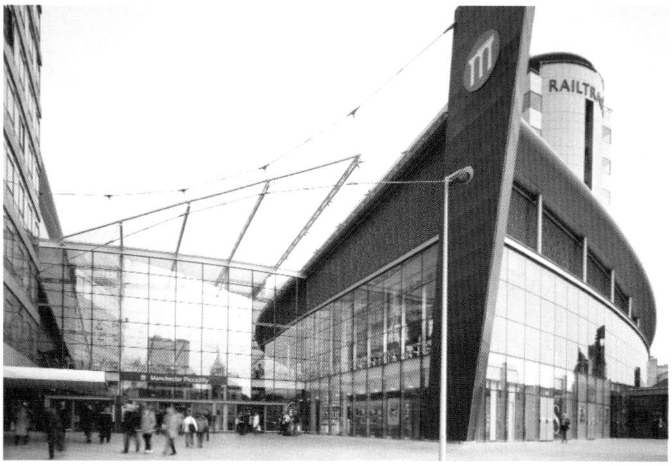

4 Manchester Piccadilly.

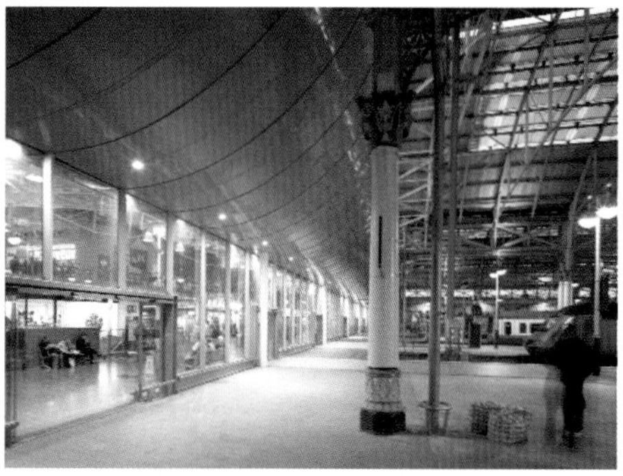

5 The platform approach.

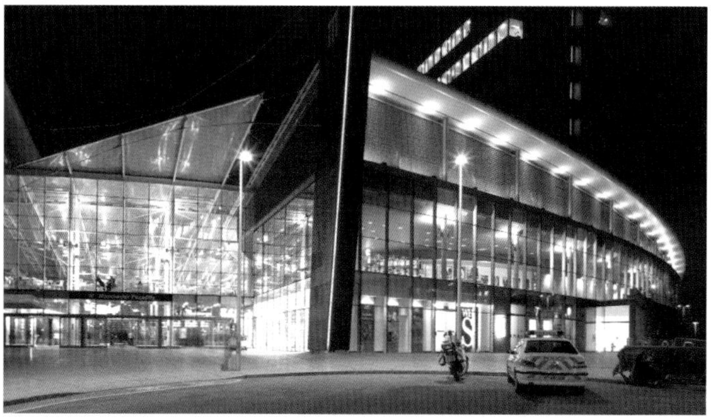

6 Drop-off point.

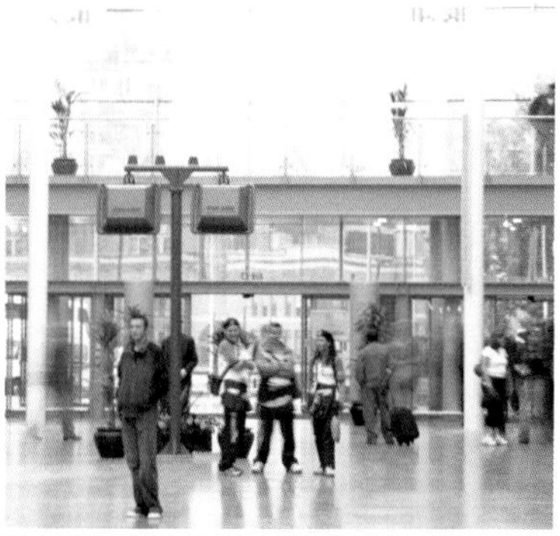

7 Pedestrian entrance.

Arrival – pedestrians

A new pedestrian entrance to Piccadilly separates pedestrian and vehicular flows, whilst taxi and private vehicles now have a dedicated drop-off/pick-up area to the south of the station on Fairfield Street.

Changes in hard landscaping use tone and texture-defined key pedestrian routes for visually impaired people. Gradients for pedestrians have been designed to meet current good practice guidelines.

Where pedestrian and vehicle routes cross, dropped kerbs or raised crossings are provided with the appropriate use of tactile blister paving. Controlled crossings have been used where appropriate.

Street furniture has been designed and located to ensure accessibility for all, including disabled children and adults.

Arrival – vehicular

The newly designed drop-of/pick-up points have been located to minimise travel distances to the station for people with walking difficulties and wheelchair users.

Suitably dimensioned accessible parking bays are located within 50 m of the building entrance and the paths between the disabled parking and drop-off/pick-up points provide level access to the station.

A number of short-stay parking spaces are provided at the station. Unfortunately these spaces, which include disabled spaces, are accessed by a barrier that is inaccessible to many disabled people. The ticketing system is also unusable by wheelchair users and people of short stature.

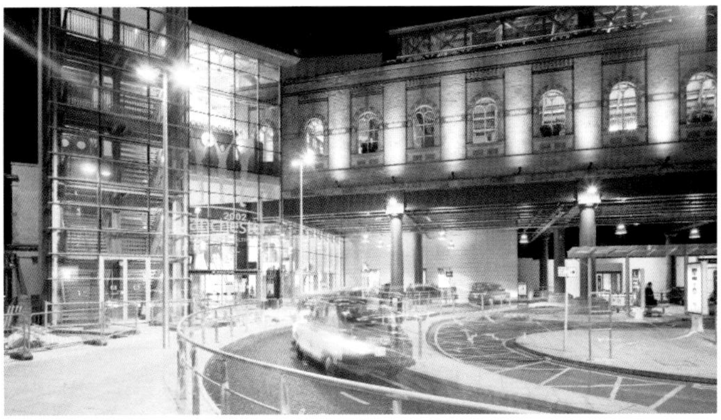

8 Short-stay parking and drop-off point.

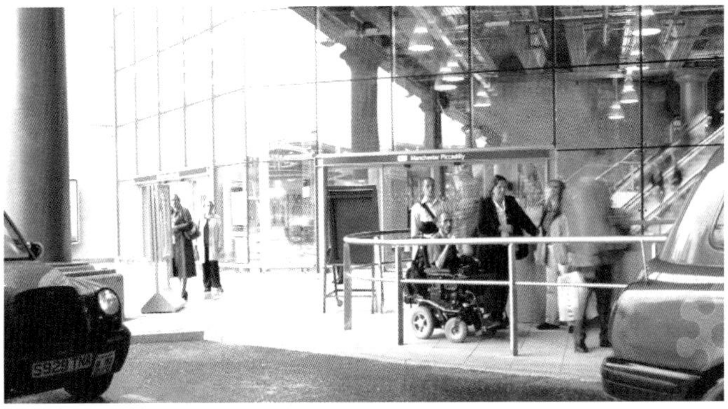

9 Taxi rank

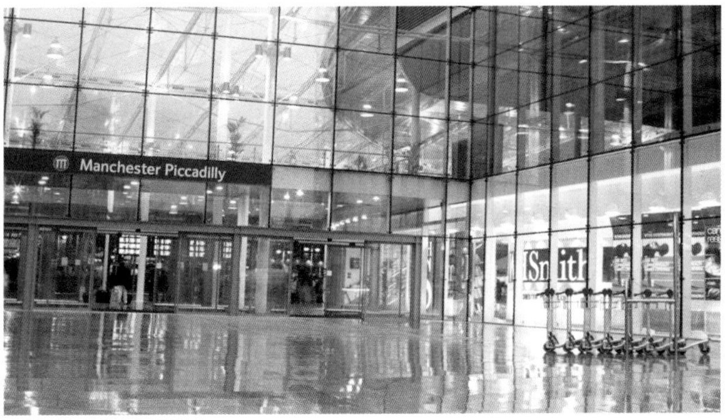

10 Entrance.

Entry

The distinct design and logical location of the principal entrances provide clear navigation aids to visitors unfamiliar with the station and have been designed to support use by disabled and visually impaired building users.

Principal entrance doors are clearly signed, contrast in luminance with their immediate surroundings and are visible in light and dark conditions.

The entrances provide level, accessible access, with flush thresholds doors. Doors have colour and tonal contrast and have suitable clear widths, allowing people using mobility aids to gain access.

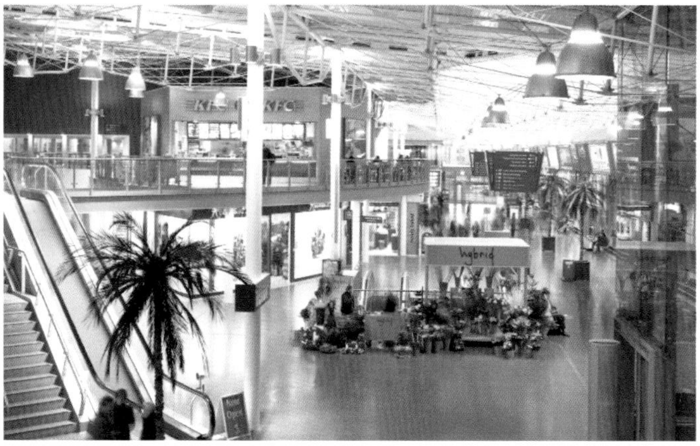

11 Concourse.

Lateral circulation

The station has been arranged in a clear and rational manner with a logical grouping of retail, travel services and platform areas.

The stairs have a continuous handrail on each side, helping people with visual or mobility impairments. Whilst the closed risers on the stairs offer advantages for accessibility, contrasting nosings should highlight each riser, but in places do not do so adequately. Lighting and finishes on the stairs are non-reflective and eliminate glare, assisting people with visual impairments.

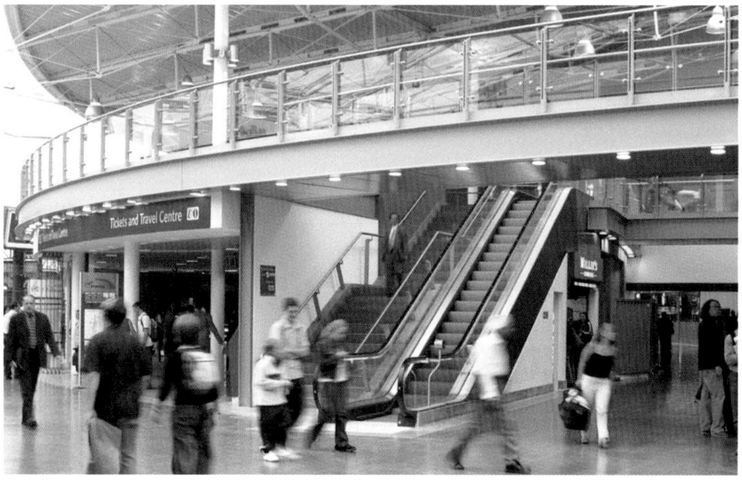

12 Stairs and escalators.

A number of lifts provide an accessible route between the upper and lower levels of the station. The lifts are supplied with emergency alarms, and are suitable for use by wheelchair users and ambulant disabled people.

The routes within the building will are a minimum width of 1800 mm wide, with main circulation routes at least 2400 mm wide.

A number of platforms at Piccadilly are located at a substantial distance from the concourse area. To help overcome these distances, moving walkways have been introduced.

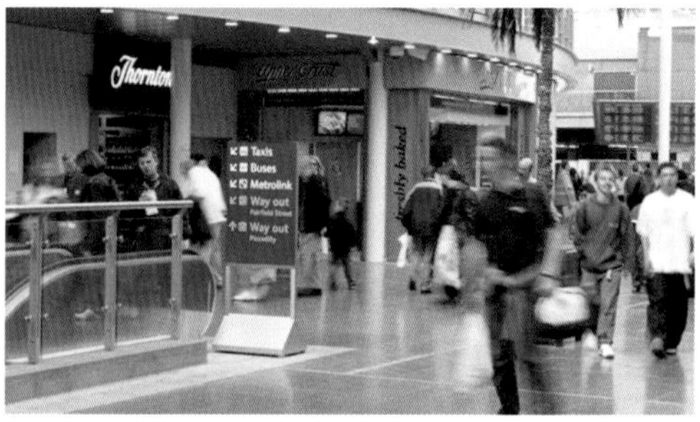

13 Movable signage.

Ticketing, information and signage

The central information point is very clearly signposted and includes low level counters for wheelchair users and people of short stature. An induction loop has been included.

Disabled people regularly make use of the assistance point, from where passengers can be helped with many aspects of their journey, from assistance with luggage, to information on ticketing for a journey. This area is very well staffed. A combination of visual and audible information is important for all users of the station, particularly for people with disabilities.

A coherent and accessible signage and information strategy is used within the station which has been designed to address the number of people travelling through the building who are be unfamiliar with the internal layout. All signage within the station has been thoughtfully designed, is accessible and functions well. The design demonstrates current good practice guidance.

Clear audible announcements are made regularly in the station, useful for people with visual impairments. The importance of providing an announcement that is significantly different in volume level to the background noise has been recognised, as has the need to repeat any announcement in this acoustically live environment.

The timetable panels have been placed adjacent to the main flow of passengers and perpendicular to circulation routes, allowing people to stand and view the information without causing an obstruction to a route; a skirting at 300 m around the base of panels allows people with a long cane to detect the obstruction.

Platforms

The platforms were refurbished between 1998 and 2000.

The platform surfaces are even, non-slip and non-reflective. A white line indicates the platform edge and a 400 mm wide tactile warning surface, which is itself set 500 mm – 700 mm from the platform edge, extends the length of the platform. This indicates the boundary of the platform for people with a visual impairment and follows guidance for the design of off-street platform paving.

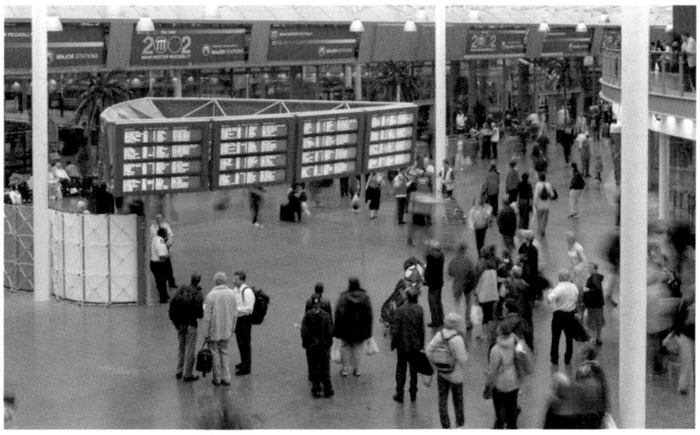

14 Information provision.

Facilities

A unisex accessible toilet which meets BS 8300: 2001 has been collocated with the standard provision on the ground floor of the building.

Seating and waiting facilities have been provided throughout the station, creating pockets of seating where people congregate, and following a more dispersed seating plan where fewer people may need to wait or rest. The design of seating follows current good practice guidelines.

15 Upper level.

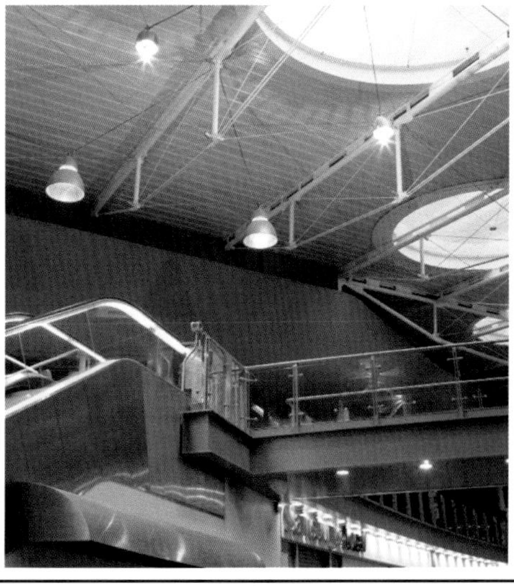

Lessons to learn

- While the journey is always the main purpose of public transport, it is the infrastructure on which that system is based which dictates the success of the system. An accessible station is an integral part of providing a transport system for all possible users.
- Although the physical environment of Piccadilly station has been designed to be accessible, continuing management of the building is essential to its remaining so. In particular, this includes the day-to-day management of audible and visual information systems, which, if removed from operation, dramatically reduce the accessibility of the station.
- The signage strategy in a large and complex building of this size and nature is crucial to making the building useable and successful. People must be able to determine where they are, and where they need to go. This need has been met successfully at Piccadilly with the introduction of a comprehensive signage strategy that demonstrates current good practice guidance.
- At Manchester the particular need to separate pedestrian and vehicular flows was recognised. It is unfortunate, however, that areas of the vehicle drop-off/pick-up points and short-stay car park have not been so carefully considered and can cause difficulties for disabled visitors, especially wheelchair users.

7.3 Newbury Town Hall

Introduction

Newbury Town Hall is located on a corner site at the junction of Mansion House Street and the Market Place, in the centre of Newbury close to the Kennet Centre shopping centre and the Kennet and Avon Canal.

The property is a Grade II listed building, constructed in the North European Gothic style. It was originally built in 1742, but was partly demolished in 1909. The current Town Hall has brick elevations under a pitched tiled roof which date back to 1910. It is arranged on three main floor levels but, with mezzanine levels, it has a total of five different floors. There are four different entrances into the building.

In general, the internal accommodation is arranged as:

Ground floor: main reception area

Second floor: Mayor's Parlour and toilets

Third floor: Council Chamber and kitchen.

There are separate office suites on the first, second and fourth floors of the building.

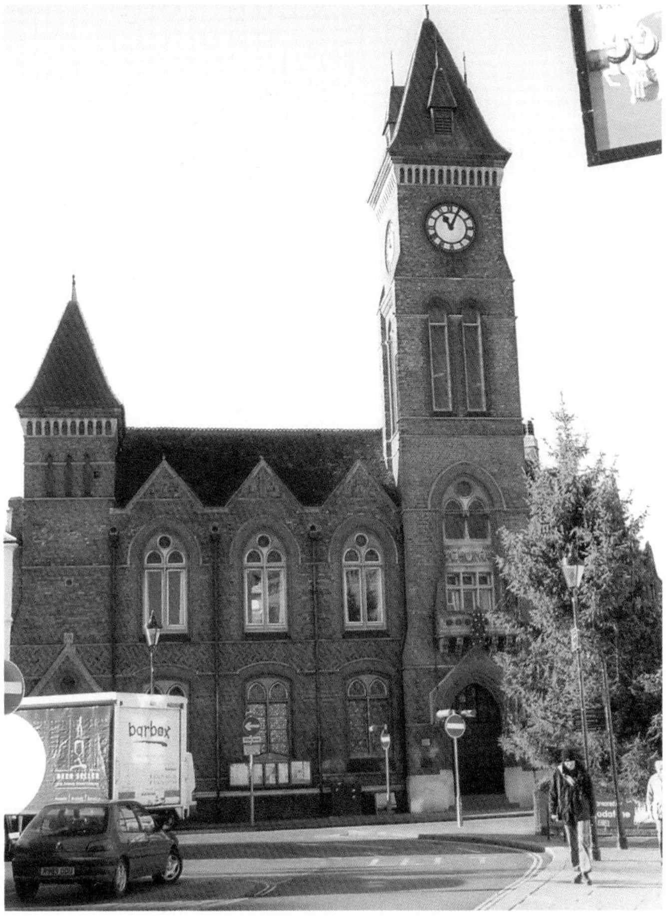

16. Newbury Town Hall viewed from the Market Place.

How the work was done

When Newbury Town Council inherited the building in 1987, the main access problems were:

- the location of the main entrance (via steps from the Market Place) which led into the main entrance lobby and impressive staircase
- the five different floor levels because of the sloping site. The main business of the Council was conducted on a half floor above the first floor, so it was particularly difficult for older people, young parents with pushchairs and other disabled people to use these facilities.
- there was no public reception area or disabled facilities.

The initial brief was to make all of the existing building accessible for everybody. In ideal circumstances, this could be achieved if there were no restrictions on costs or the type of work that could be carried out. However, the special architectural and historical significance of this building placed obvious constraints on the type of work that would be permitted by the local authority. There were also constraints imposed by the amount of funding that could be made available for any access work. In this example, the sources of funding included the Public Works Loans Board, the Council's Earmarked Capital Project Reserves and General Reserves, and a grant from the local authority. The total amount was approximately £207 000.

Initially, a proposal was put forward to install an attendant-operated wheelchair lift – from the original entrance in the Market Place to the ground floor entrance lobby – with a stairlift fitted to the main staircase leading to the first floor and the half landing on the same floor as the Council Chamber. This would have provided access to the Council Chamber only, and would not have made other areas of the building accessible. Also, the visual impact of a stairlift on the imposing staircase would have significantly altered the overall appearance of one of the main architectural features of the building.

This proposal was later refined to include the installation of a purpose-built platform lift which would provide access to all five floor levels of the building including the Council offices, the Mayor's Parlour and the Council Chamber. Other proposed work included:

- changing the location of the main entrance to the side entrance in Mansion House Street and installing railings outside this entrance
- providing an induction loop in the proposed reception area adjoining the Council Chamber
- providing accessible toilet facilities
- creating a new landing on the third floor to allow access from the lift to the Council Chamber.

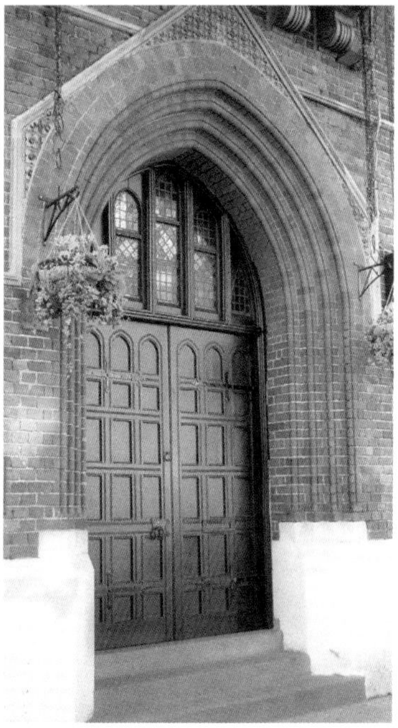

17 Original entrance, with three steps, viewed from the Market Place.

Plans were submitted for the proposed work and Building Regulations and Listed Building Consent were obtained in autumn 2000.

Before any work was carried out, the existing office tenants had to be relocated. The original electrical switchgear was repositioned and the new lift shaft and platform lift were installed. The new reception area was created just inside the new main entrance, the new landing was built on the third floor adjoining the Council Chamber. The accessible toilet facilities were created on the second floor. The final phase of the work was to relocate the main council offices to the ground floor and automate the existing doors to the new main entrance.

Car parking and approach

There is no allocated car parking provided at the Town Hall, but most of the public car parks in the centre of Newbury incorporate accessible spaces. The approach to the building is via the various pedestrian footpaths which lead from these car parks to the Town Hall.

Entry

There are four entrances into the building: one from Bartholomew Street, one from Mansion House Street which was previously used as a fire exit, and two from the Market Place. The original main entrance was from the Market Place but part of the access improvements included realigning the footpath in Mansion House Street to eliminate the existing step at the entrance on this side of the building.

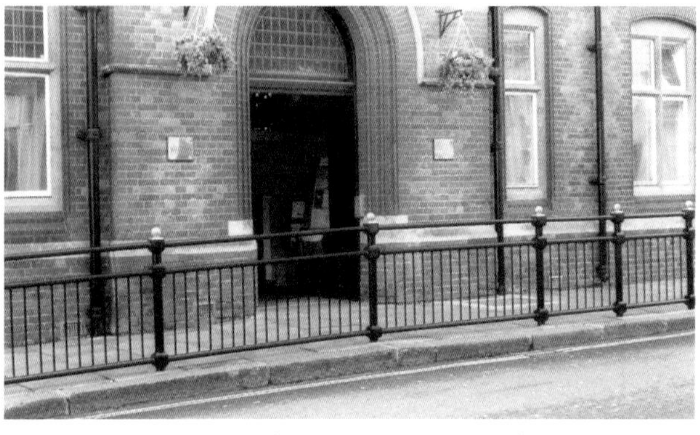

18 New main entrance from Mansion House Street showing level entrance and pedestrian railings.

This entrance is now used as the new main entrance into the building. The original main entrance in the Market Place is still used for some events, but the signage indicates that all visitors should use the entrance in Mansion House Street. The main reception area is located immediately inside this entrance, from which all visitors can be directed to different parts of the Town Hall. An induction loop has been installed to assist hearing-impaired visitors. The new entrance has meant that disabled visitors do not have to use a separate entrance, and any work that has been carried out has been done in sympathy with the existing building. The new main entrance has been protected from the street with a pedestrian railing located at the edge of the footpath.

Horizontal circulation

Work carried out to assist horizontal circulation around the building has included the fitting of new door closers to the internal doors at the original main entrance. This has meant that the double doors now open into the entrance hallway rather than into the lobby at the bottom of the main impressive staircase. This is a good example of how the latest type of technology has been incorporated into an existing historical building.

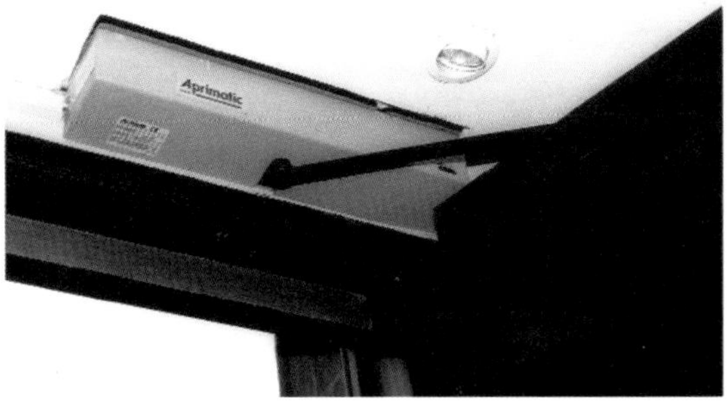

19. Door closer fitted to double doors.

On the third floor, a new landing has been created, immediately outside the Council Chamber, which has made this section of the building accessible for all users. The work has been carried out in sympathy with the original character and layout of the building. All visitors can now use the Council Chamber when attending functions at the Town Hall.

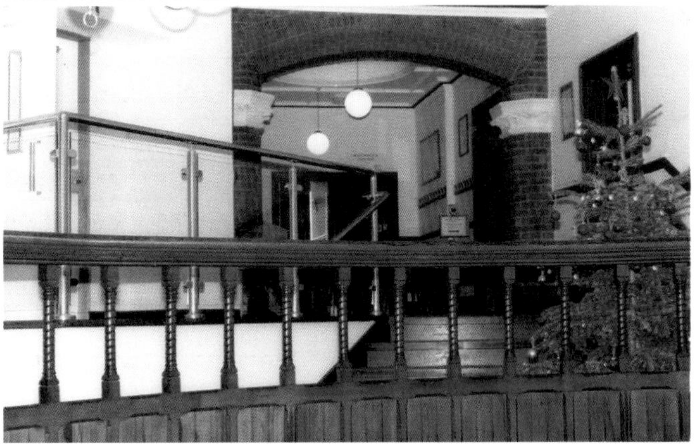

20 New landing constructed outside lift (left) providing access to the Council Chamber (far right).

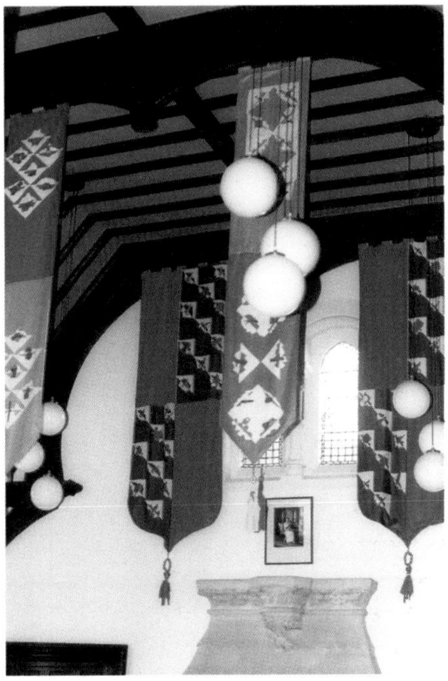

21 The ceiling of the Council Chamber.

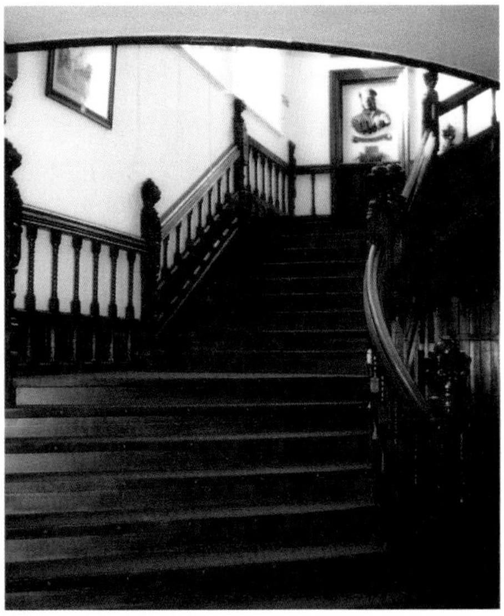

22 The main staircase.

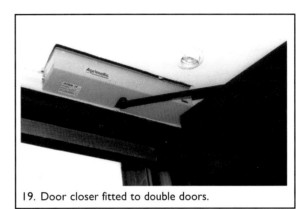

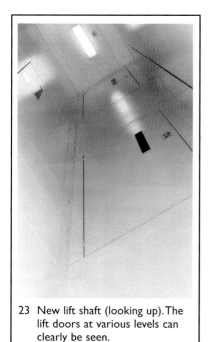

Vertical circulation

One of the main access problems with the existing building was the number of intermediate changes of floor level and the need to protect the architectural character and integrity of the imposing main staircase. This problem was addressed by installing a lift into a new vertical shaft away from the main staircase area but which provided access to all five floor levels of the building. This work did not dramatically change the existing floor layout but opened up other areas of the building that were previously inaccessible.

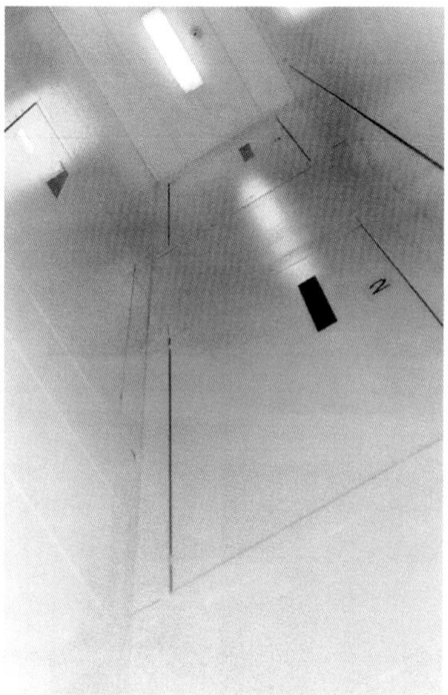
23 New lift shaft (looking up). The lift doors at various levels can clearly be seen.

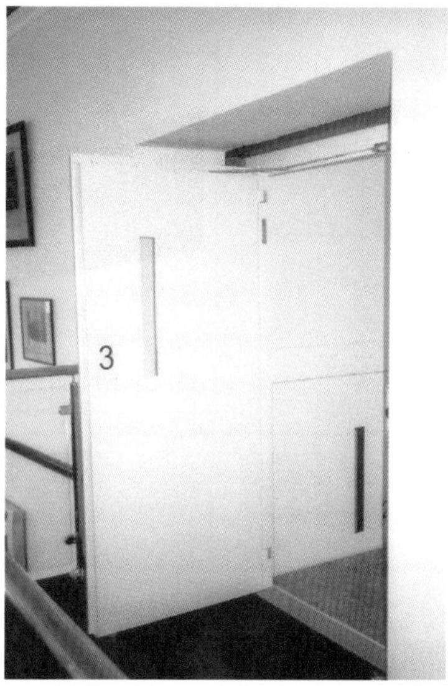
3
24 The lift door leading on the new landing created by Council Chamber. The lift door to level 2 of the building can be seen in the lift shaft.

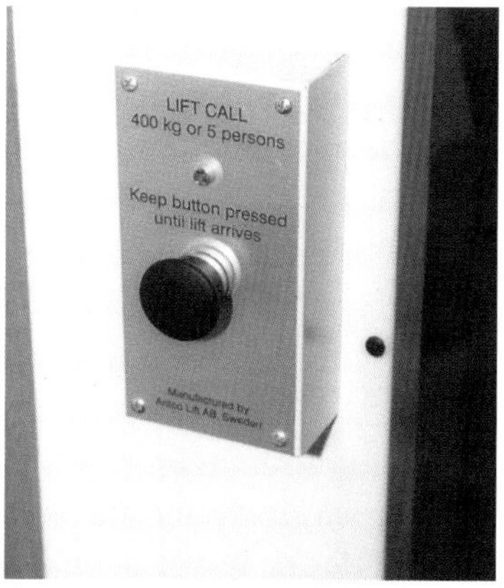
LIFT CALL
400 kg or 5 persons
Keep button pressed
until lift arrives
25 The lift call button.

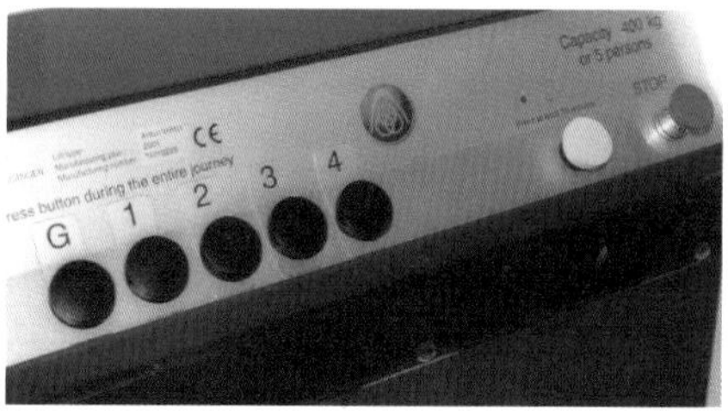

26 The lift control buttons.

Facilities

Accessible toilet facilities have been created on the second floor in close proximity to the lift, which makes them easier to use from all areas of the building. Good colour contrast has been incorporated between the sanitary fittings and their tiled background and the door ironmongery is well contrasted and easy to grip. An emergency pull cord has been installed which, when activated, illuminates a sign in the lobby adjoining the lift.

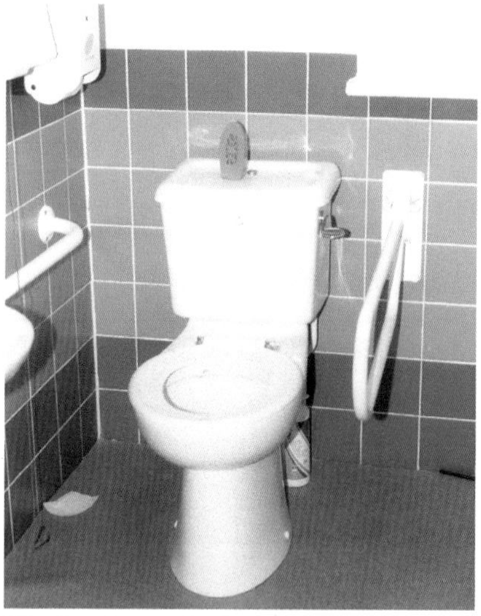
27 Good use of colour and luminance contrast.

Lessons to learn

- It is important to consult as many relevant parties as possible on issues relating to access. In this case study, input was obtained from the West Berkshire liaison group on disability and other local disabled people.
- Even if an existing building is listed, there are usually solutions to access problems that do not significantly alter the existing fabric and structure. The only change to the external appearance of the building in this case study has been the introduction of two brass plaques and a control panel immediately adjacent to the newly automated doors at the new main entrance in Mansion House Street.
- It is important to phase access work in an existing building. In this example, it was important that the existing tenants were relocated before any access work started.

Benefits

The main benefit of carrying out this access work has been that all disabled people, including those who use a larger than average size wheelchair, can use all areas of the building, including the Mayor's Parlour and the Council Chamber for the first time in the history of the Town Hall.

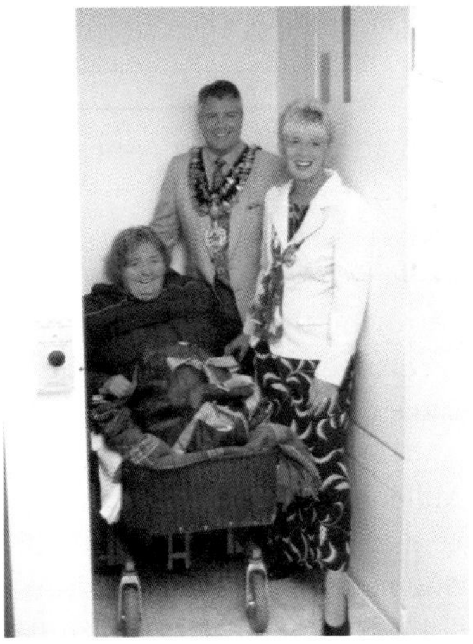

28 Using the lift.

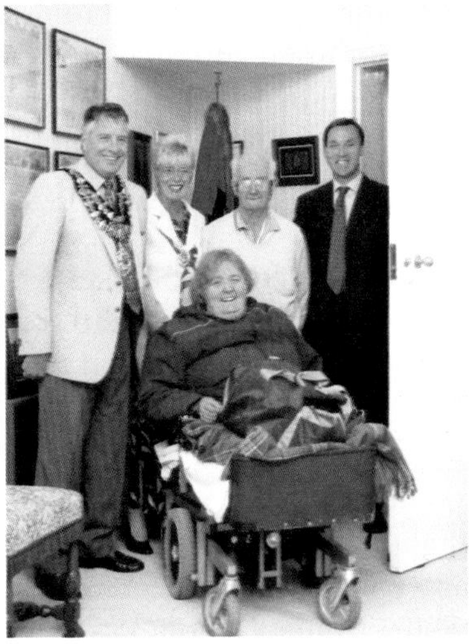

29 Into the Mayor's Parlour.

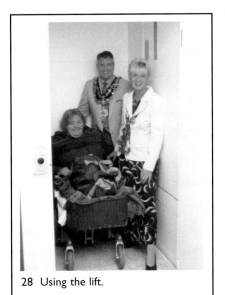

7.4 St Mary's Church, Kintbury, Berkshire

Introduction

St Mary's Church is situated within the village of Kintbury, approximately four miles west of Newbury, Berkshire. Originally, a Saxon church occupied this site, but the current church – parts of which date back to the 11th century – later replaced it. Further additions were carried out in the 14th and 18th centuries. The church is constructed of stone and brick, and the square tower at the western end of the church has recently been repaired and redecorated.

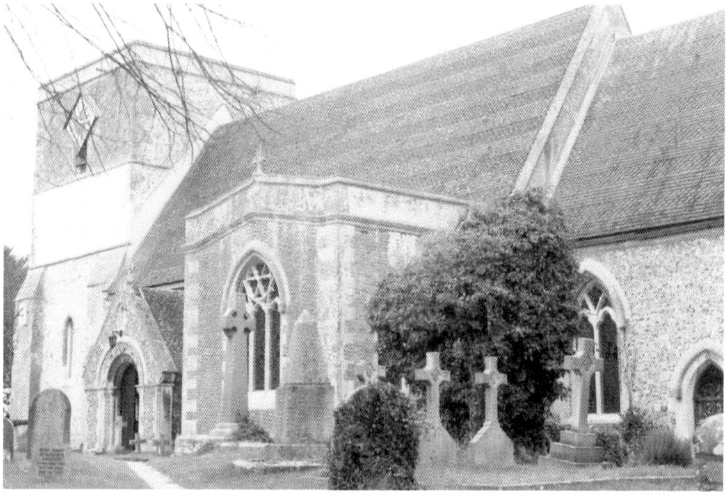

30 St Mary's Church, Kintbury (south elevation).

A church, because of its historic significance, often presents many challenges in terms of access issues. This case study has been used to illustrate ways in which some of these issues can be addressed, and offer encouragement to individuals and organisations who may need to address similar issues and problems when considering inclusive access.

As with many older buildings, especially churches, accessibility had always been an issue at St Mary's. However, the need to consider improving the access to the church was highlighted when one parishioner, who had developed a relatively rapid degenerative condition, was prevented from marrying in the church because it did not meet her access needs.

In response to this, the church started its "Millennium Challenge", which was to establish accessibility to both the church and its adjacent hall for the new Millennium. In 1998, an access committee was formed, whose members included the priest, senior church officials and parishioners, one of whom was an architect. Their brief was to steer and coordinate all work related to accessibility issues and ensure liaison with other church committees and local organisations.

In one creative move, contact was made with the local University, and this brought about the involvement of the Research Group for Inclusive Environments (RGIE) at The University of Reading. Following an initial visit, undergraduate students undertook a supervised access audit of the church and the adjoining hall. This work contributed as coursework for the students taking a final year Inclusive Environments Option as part of their studies in building surveying. The students presented their findings and recommendations to members of the St Mary's access committee.

Car parking

The access audit identified inappropriate car parking for disabled people, both in terms of the numbers of places provided and their distance from the church. There were no designated parking spaces for disabled people and no safe areas identified on the adjoining road to assist safe movement to the church. The surface of the parking area was uneven and in poor repair, and partly obstructed by large refuse bins.

A suggested recommendation, subject to the necessary permission, was to convert the grassed area immediately outside the west door into an area suitable for disabled parking and as a drop-off area. The plan is for a hard standing to allow three designated parking bays for disabled people and a drop-off point. Access to this area will be via the track between the south gate and the north gate, which is wide enough for a car.

Approach

The existing gravel paths were identified as being a problem for wheelchair users. Other pathways were uneven and gaps between existing floor slabs created tripping hazards. Some of the existing paved surfaces were slippery in wet weather. Narrow pathways, a small step (150 mm high) on the path from the east gate to the main entrance, and the lengthy approach between the road and main entrance all presented problems, particularly for wheelchair users and people using mobility aids. Money has been raised to resurface one of the paths and there are plans to upgrade or replace the other paths to the south and west doors, where applicable.

The access committee recognised the lack of any good external lighting around the church as a particular problem for visitors and members of the congregation, especially those with poor vision, when using paths across the churchyard at night. However, any improvements had to ensure that the historical and aesthetic integrity of the church was not compromised in any way.

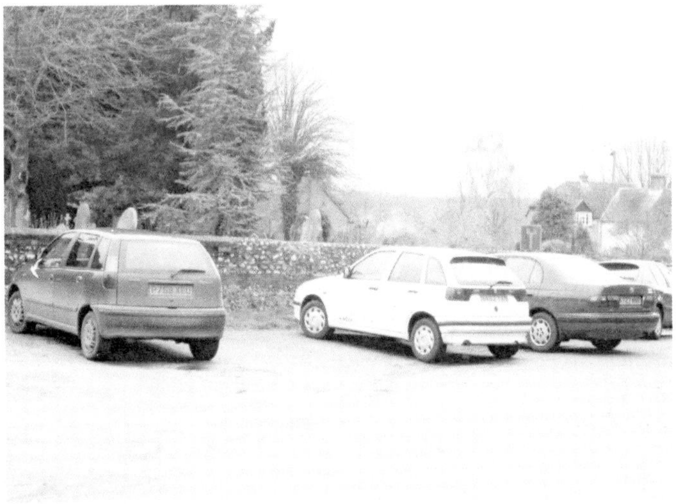

31 On-street car parking.

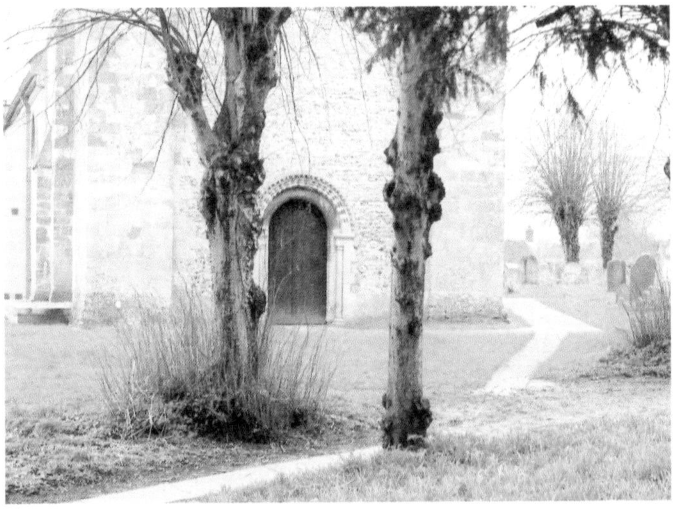

32 A potential area for accessible car parking bays by the west door.

33 Loose gravel paths that are difficult for many disabled people to negotiate.

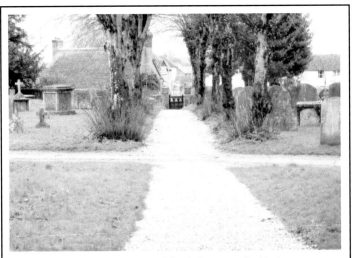

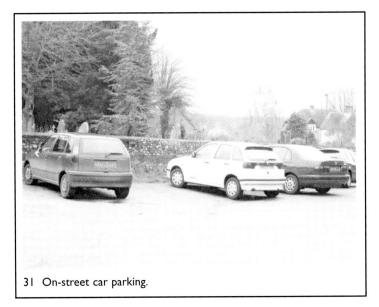

Two systems of lighting were considered:

- a system which illuminated the churchyard by the installation of, for example, lamp standards
- a low level system of bollard lighting to highlight pathways and provide general way guidance information.

It was decided that the second system would be the most appropriate and bollard light fittings will be provided to highlight pathways and give directional way-guiding information.

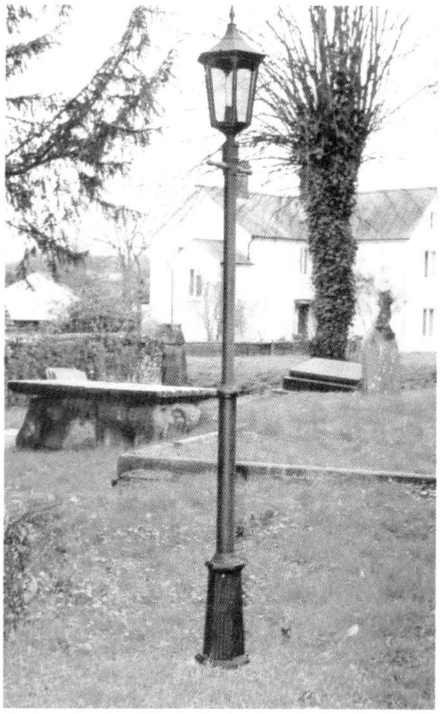

34 An example of the existing lighting to the churchyard, which was poor.

Entry

The small step with two further steps into the church was difficult for wheelchair users at the south gate entrance. At the west door entrance, there was a step down into the foyer which, again, was difficult for someone in a wheelchair.

There was no real prospect of providing an internal ramp inside the church that would be either visually or spatially acceptable. Also, unlike other public access buildings where planning permission or building regulations are required for substantial improvements, approval for any church improvements is required from the diocese. Any such work has to be carried out in keeping with the architectural and historical interest of the church, and it was unlikely that providing an internal ramp would satisfy these conditions. It is very unlikely that any work which compromised the historical importance of the double doors giving access into the main body of the church from the porch, would have been approved.

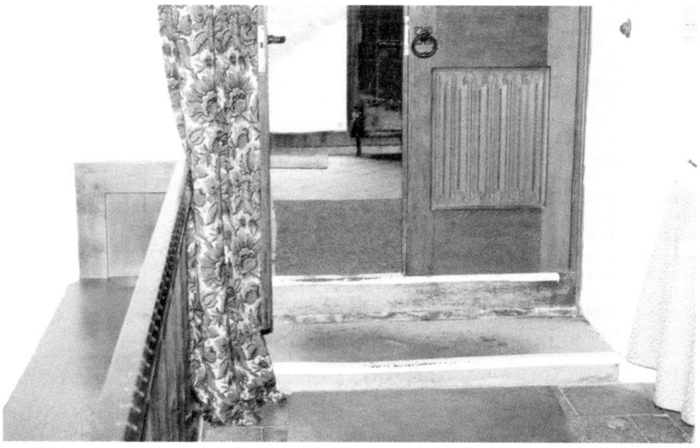

35 Restricted access that was impossible to overcome internally.

Lateral circulation

Since the access audit, the flooring inside the west entrance porch has been raised by approximately 60 mm up to the same level as the present height of the existing step. This has created a flat access route inside the church, which is particularly beneficial for wheelchair users and people with mobility impairments.

Also, the space between the font and the last row of pews was originally too narrow for a wheelchair user. This has been improved by shortening one of the rear pews by approximately 500 mm and creating space for wheelchair users to approach the font.

Services

At the time of the access audit, it was difficult for a person with a hearing impairment to lip-read the speaker in the pulpit as it was positioned so that the priest's face was obstructed. Since then, an induction loop has been provided which has assisted people with hearing impairments to listen to sermons and lectures. Other improvements have been introduced to assist visually impaired people, including the provision of large print information and hymn sheets.

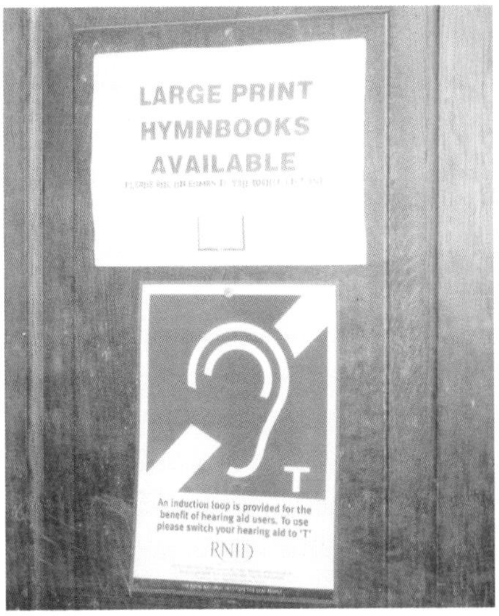

36 Access to information is equally as important as access to the church. Unfortunately the printed sign is temporary and in upper case only, which is not best practice.

Facilities

The provision of accessible toilet facilities was an issue of particular concern to the access committee. The inadequacy of existing toilet accommodation is a common problem not just for churches, but for many other community buildings, such as church halls, village halls and community centres.

When the access audit was originally carried out, no accessible toilet facilities existed. The only toilet accommodation was located in the hall adjoining the church, referred to as St Mary's Hall, where space was restricted in and around the toilet cubicles and there was a lack of colour contrast between the walls and fittings. Increasing the size of the hall to accommodate new toilet facilities was not an option.

One way of addressing this problem was to redesign the existing layout by introducing, within the existing spaces, the use of the unisex facilities. This course of action was considered to be the most appropriate. On behalf of the access committee, RGIE designed the proposed improvement work that involved refurbishing the existing male and female toilet facilities (one WC cubicle, one urinal and one hand basin in the male toilet and one WC cubicle and one hand basin in the female), to provide two unisex accessible toilets each containing:

- an accessible WC
- a urinal
- two hand basins (one positioned at a height that was accessible from the WC),
- baby changing facilities.

The new layouts of these facilities allowed for a choice of both right and left hand transfer to be provided. This refurbishment work illustrates how various options and an increased number of choices can be provided within the same space. The new configurations have ensured that there are facilities available for disabled and non-disabled, female and male members of the public. This was achieved within the original space and without altering the original location of the toilets.

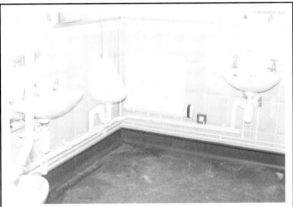

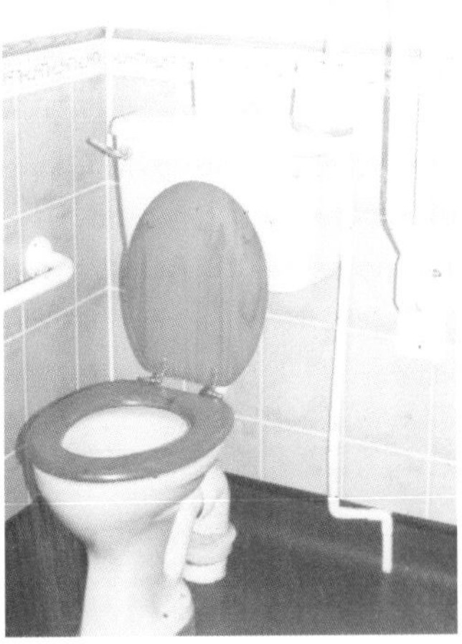

37 & 38 Two accessible toilets, one providing left-hand transfer and the other right-hand transfer, replace the existing male and female toilets. Each toilet is fitted with a urinal and wash hand basins. They are suitable for both disabled and non-disabled people. Two unisex toilets provide full facilities without the need to increase the space available, and the contrast has been achieved at no additional cost.

The new toilet accommodation was decorated using good colour contrast between the sanitary fittings and their background, and the lighting level was improved with good light fittings. Good colour contrast and improved lighting are examples of improvements that can be carried out inexpensively and at any time within an existing building. In this example, this work was done at the date of refurbishment, but it could also have been done as part of an ongoing maintenance and management schedule of work.

How the work was done

The formation of the access committee in 1998 acted as a driving force for access work at the church. Involving people who were familiar with the existing layout of the building, and listening to their own personal experiences and problems of gaining access into the church and moving around inside it, allowed constructive, practical decisions to be made.

Access committees, such as the one at St Mary's, rely very much upon voluntary contributions by their members. In this particular example, the committee was fortunate to have one member who was a qualified architect and was happy to share his professional expertise without charging a fee.

Being able to use the suggestions provided by the students and members of RGIE, rather than professional organisations such as access consultants, architects, surveyors and occupational therapists, has also helped to eliminate the need for consultancy fees. However, this was a partnership in which the access committee achieved its goals, the students were able to experience how to address the needs of a real client creatively, and many of the findings of the research work undertaken by RGIE could be applied further in practice.

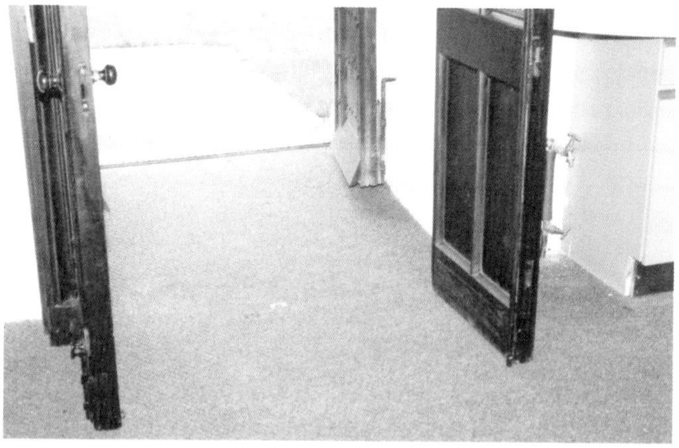

39 A small step down into the area inside the west door was addressed by raising the floor. This also addressed the small step up into the main body of the church, creating a level entrance and route directly into the church.

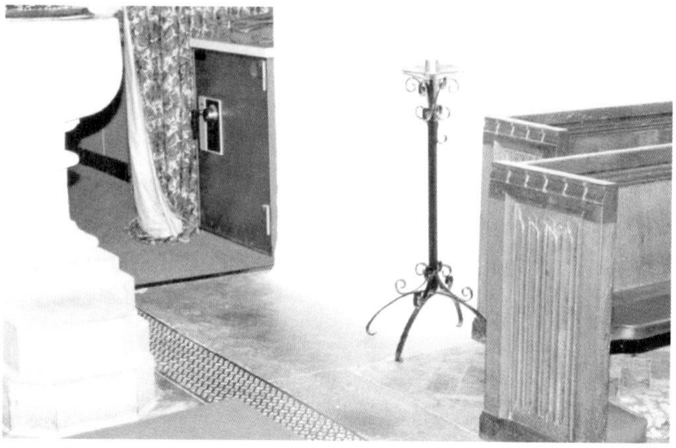

40 The distance between the font and the rear pew obstructed access through the church from the west door. Moving the font was not possible. Re-aligning the rear pew has now enabled full access. A few management issues – like the placing of the candle holder – need addressing, but it was a good solution to a difficult problem.

Lessons to learn

- Always listen to personal experiences of people using the building, if they are available and relevant. People are very happy to volunteer for committees if they feel that other people are listening to and acting upon their suggestions.
- Make use of any relevant professionally trained people if they are happy to provide their own expertise at minimal or no cost.
- Look to other organisations such as universities and other educational establishments, local voluntary bodies etc for input.
- Recognise that access improvement work does not always have to cost a large amount of money – some improvements can be carried out with the minimum of disturbance and cost and can be included within existing maintenance and management programmes. This can be illustrated in the improved colour contrast and lighting in the new unisex accessible toilet accommodation.
- Always clarify at the outset what permissions are required for any alterations or improvements to avoid unnecessary reworking and time delays.
- It is important to design for as wide an environment as possible – inclusive design is the key. The toilets in this case study illustrate good design for everyone.
- There is more that one solution to a particular access problem. The different types of exterior lighting referred to in the case study illustrate two options for improving external lighting.
- Access work takes time, so establishing priorities for different work is important. In the case study, the access committee identified entry into the church, using the services within the church and the existing toilet as the most important problems to address at an early stage.
- If the building is of significant architectural and/or historical significance, compromises have to be made regarding access issues. It is not possible to do everything and some recommendations cannot be carried out because of existing constructional details or the need to conserve existing artefacts, etc.

Part two – design guidance

8 External approach

The accessibility of the approach to a building or environment is as important as the level of accessibility within it. This chapter considers the issues which can affect independent and, importantly, safe external access.

8.1 Design principles

8.1.1 Convenient vehicle access

Setting down points and parking should be as close as possible to accessible entrances. Enough space should be allowed for loading and unloading wheelchairs and other equipment. A management procedure should be instigated to ensure that other users do not block setting down points and parking for disabled people.

See 8.5

8.1.2 Short, safe, level routes

Pedestrian routes for disabled people should be short, level and easy to negotiate. The need to cross and share vehicle routes should be avoided as far as possible. Direct access to the entrance of the building is important for everyone. It is much harder for a wheelchair user or someone with a mobility impairment to cover the distance from the car park or nearest transport link than it is for a non-disabled person. Gradients, steps and surfaces all need to meet best practice guidelines.

8.1.3 Well-signposted routes

Accessible entrances should be clearly signposted from all access points, including car parking, transport links and setting down points. It is particularly frustrating and unnecessary for people with mobility impairments to have to retrace the path after taking a wrong turning owing to poor signage. Clear directional signage that is well-positioned and consistent, benefits all users.

8.1.4 One route for all

The same pedestrian approach routes should, whenever possible, be accessible for all users. It is not acceptable for disabled people to have to use a different route from any non-disabled companions or non-disabled people in general.

See 9.1, 8.2.2

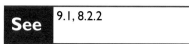

8.1.5 Accessible controls

Controls and security systems should be designed so that they are easy to use and positioned in an accessible location. Unintentional barriers can be created for people with disabilities, such as having to speak into an intercom or turn a small knob to gain entry into a building. Designers should select equipment and specify its location to meet the needs of all users.

See 8.5.1

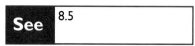

8.2 Strategy for existing buildings

8.2.1 Improving access routes

The accessibility of both external and internal routes is crucial. Equal rights of access should be available to all users wherever reasonably practicable. It is essential to address the inherent problems imposed by the site for disabled people, in conjunction with improvements to the building itself.

Improvements that make the approach to a building easier for disabled people to manage are not always immediately obvious. Gate controls or ticket machines for the car parking area may be difficult to operate, or it may be just that traffic lights on a crossing change too quickly to allow a person who has difficulty walking to cross safely. Management procedures such as reserving a car parking space immediately in front of a building, or having permission to park in the forecourt of an nearby property, can influence greatly the accessibility of an environment.

8.2.2 Avoiding a separate access route

A separate route for disabled people to access a building should be avoided wherever possible, as all users should have an equal right to access. If this is unavoidable in certain situations, the best course of action may be to redirect everyone onto a separate route that bypasses obstacles such as steps, slopes and unsuitable surfaces, rather than provide a separate route for disabled people.

Where the internal planning of the building allows, it may be possible to change the principal entrance to one that is accessible. Where the main entrance to the building is not the accessible entrance, particular care will be needed with signposting. It is essential that the accessible entrance is not the "back entrance" to the building or seen to be of an inferior standard to the main entrance.

8.2.3 Overcoming site restraints

Existing sites can present many constraints and the scope for physically rearranging them is usually limited by space, gradients, conservation issues and cost:

- existing steps, kerbs, parking control systems and gates and railings may all present difficulties – an access audit should prioritise improvements
- the best routes to accessible entrances from setting down points, car parking and public transport, may not be easy to find – the use of clear, consistent, directional signage is essential to orientate all building users
- paths and parking areas may have unsuitable surfaces such as cobbles or loose gravel – stabilisation and rolling a binder into the gravel may be a solution
- there may be no space for any parking – a solution may be to instigate a management procedure to allocate space for disabled parking or a drop-off point
- if the only alternative to steep slopes and steps is a long circuitous route, or if the car parking is a considerable distance from the entrance, it may be possible to provide an alternative site access or alternative parking for disabled people
- landscaping may obstruct potential parking areas and should be reviewed.

8.2.4 Management procedures

The instigation of management procedures to assist disabled people can eliminate barriers to accessing a building.

Examples of management procedures are:

- using gates that are normally closed
- having cars parked by an attendant
- ensuring that accessible car parking spaces are used by Blue Badge holders only.

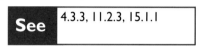

See 4.3.3, 11.2.3, 15.1.1

8.3 Setting down points

8.3.1 Safety, convenience and ease of use

The location, space allocated and adjacent details of setting down points can be critical for disabled people, and in general should:

- be provided in addition to allocated accessible parking bays
- be as close as possible to the entrance
- have a level surface
- have adequate length and width for the unloading of wheelchairs and equipment
- have dropped kerbs to give access to adjacent pavements
- be well lit
- provide shelter whenever possible.

8.3.2 Location

Setting down and collection is an essential issue with regard to accessing a building. Discussion with the Highways Authority is advisable to ensure highway policies do not conflict with improvements in the accessibility of the building. The Authority may be able to provide a marked stopping area or bay on the highway.

More than one setting down point may be required if more than one entrance is used by disabled people. The location of taxi ranks, bus stops, and waiting spaces for cars should also be convenient for entrances and exits used by disabled people.

8.3.3 Appropriate size

Space should be provided at the side and either end of the space to allow for the unloading of wheelchairs and equipment and for transferring safely in/out of the vehicle to/from a wheelchair.

8.3.4 Management procedure

A setting down point for disabled people close to a main entrance is likely to be used by everyone. A management procedure should be instigated to control the space and ensure it is available exclusively for disabled people (see also Chapter 4).

8.3.5 Providing shelter

Providing a shelter over setting down points is recommended where feasible. Many site constraints would prevent this, such as conservation issues, structural restrictions, or cost.

See 9.1.5

8.4 Parking

8.4.1 Convenience

The location, the way it is controlled and how parking is detailed, are all issues that affect the convenience and usability of parking facilities.

Car parking should:

- be easily identifiable with clear and consistent directional signage
- should, if appropriate, be available both for employees and visitors
- have designated accessible parking bays as close to the entrance as possible
- meet the dimensions as recommended in BS 8300: 2001
- be level and next to firm, even and slip-resistant pedestrian surfaces
- have dropped kerbs to give access to adjacent pavements
- be well lit
- have entry controls that are easy to use by everyone.

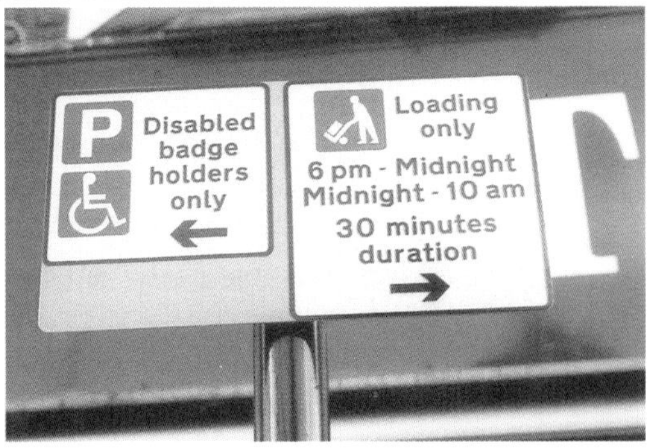
P
Disabled badge holders only
←
Loading only
6 pm - Midnight
Midnight - 10 am
30 minutes duration
→

1. Parking bays for disabled people (Blue Badge holders) should be clearly identified from other parking areas.

8.4.2 Location and provision

When space and access conditions allow, accessible designated parking bays should be provided close to the main entrance. Information regarding the vertical clearance should be provided at the entrance to some car parks to inform drivers of any height restrictions for high top converted vehicles. In addition, information regarding payment should also be provided at the entrance to car parks to make it clear to all motorists whether or not payment is required. Many car parking facilities provide free parking for disabled people who are Blue Badge holders.

On sites which slope steeply it is important to place the accessible parking bays in the most convenient position for disabled employees or visitors to use. If possible, accessible parking bays should be provided where the slope is at same level as the entrance.

It is recommended that parking for disabled people should not be more than 50 m from the entrance to the building (100 m if the route is covered). Where designated accessible parking bays are provided for Blue Badge holders, it is also recommended that some consideration is given to people who do not qualify because their impairments are less severe or temporary, but who still experience difficulty walking a long distance from the car park. In many circumstances, this issue can be controlled with the instigation of a management procedure.

The number of allocated accessible parking places provided should be appropriate for the type and use of building that they serve. The following specific guidelines are given in BS 8300: 2001 for the number of such spaces. However, an access audit should determine the requirement for allocated accessible parking bays in each individual case.

- **Workplaces** – one space for each disabled employee plus two per cent of the total capacity for visitors (minumum one space). For unknown numbers of disabled employees, five per cent of total capacity
- **Shopping centres and leisure facilities** – one for each disabled employee plus six per cent of total capacity
- **Railway stations** – one for each disabled employee plus five per cent total capacity
- **Churches/crematoria** – at least two spaces.

8.4.3 Dimensions and markings

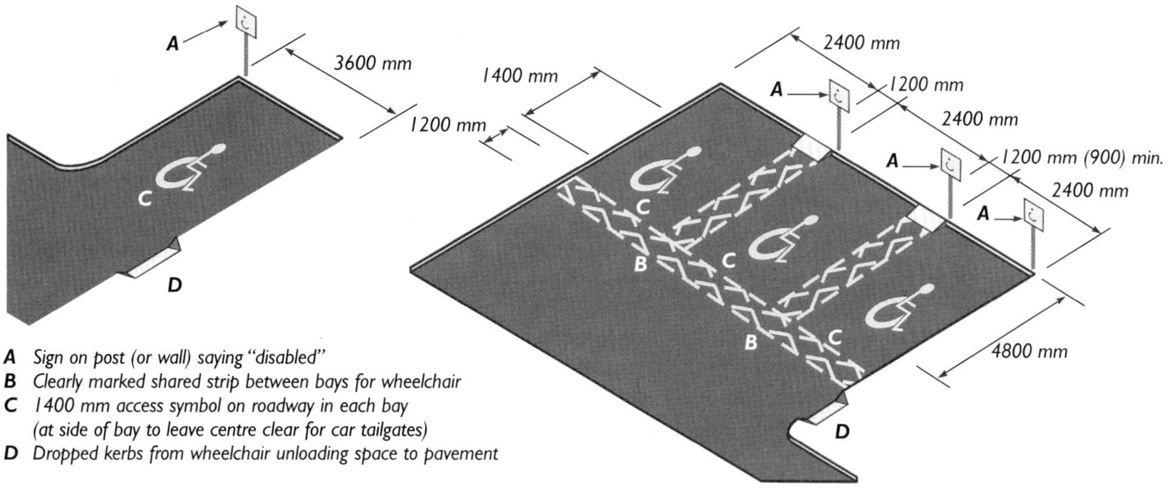

Figure 8a Off-street designated accessible parking bays should be 2400 mm x 4800 mm with a 1200 mm safety zone, which should be clearly identified with hatched markings around one side of the bay and the rear, to allow disabled motorists to get out of the vehicle, unload equipment and manoeuvre safely between other parked cars.

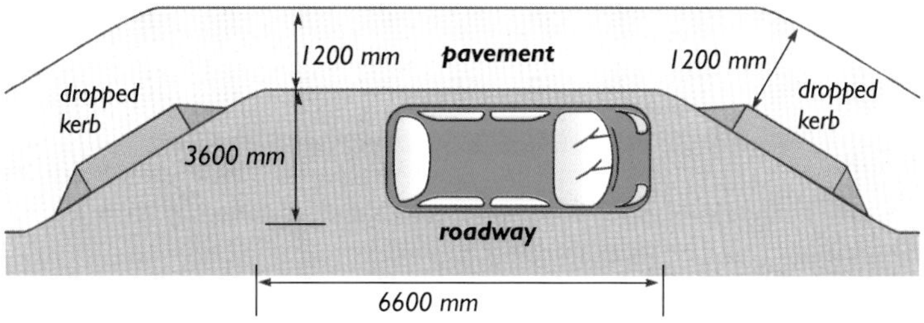

Figure 8b On-street designated accessible bays should be 6600 mm x 3600 mm (which incorporates safety transfer zones at the side and rear of the vehicle) with suitable dropped kerbs.

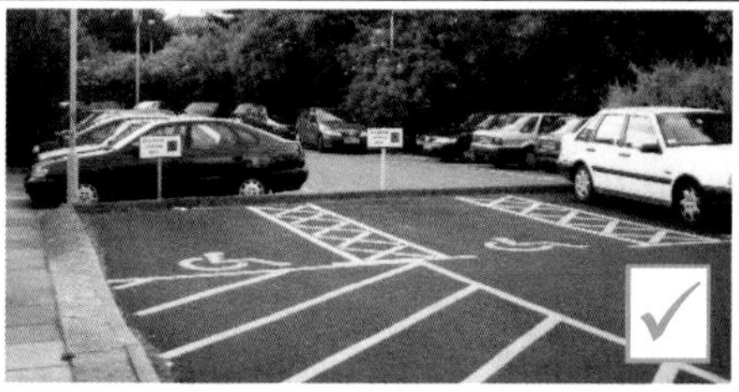

2. Good, clear, surface marking. The vertical signs at the head of the bays should be higher so they are visible above any cars parked in the bays.

Surface markings of allocated accessible bays may be obscured by snow, mud or fallen leaves and so upright signs displaying the access symbol should be provided at the head of each bay (off street parking only). In addition it is recommended that a 1400 mm access symbol is clearly marked on the surface of every bay.

8.4.4 Surfaces

All parking bay surfaces should be smooth, level and slip-resistent. Maintenance of car parking areas should be ongoing to keep them free from debris and standing water (reducing hazards for disabled people) and to keep markings and signage clear from obstructions.

The preferred types of parking surfaces for wheelchair users are not always acceptable within historic environments. A compromise may be possible by providing pathways between bays using flagstones or light coloured stone aggregate paving with an epoxy binder.

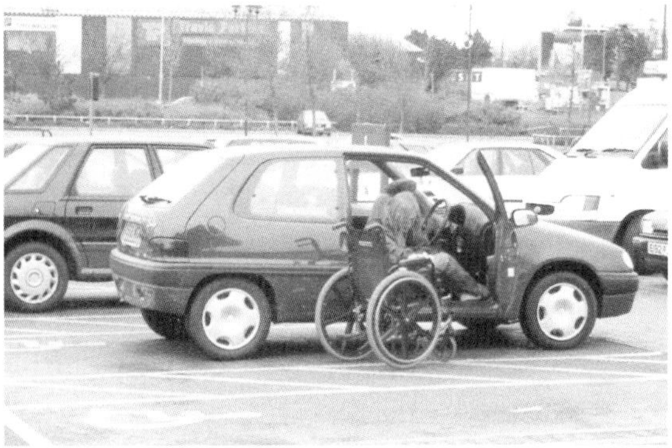

3. The area for transfer is clearly marked at the sides of the bay. There is no marking at the end of the bay but there is sufficient space to exit a car without using the circulation routes.

8.5 Vehicle access controls

8.5.1 Accessible controls

Vehicle access controls should create neither a barrier, preventing access for disabled people, nor unnecessary difficulties for disabled people operating the controls:

- disabled people should never have to exit their cars to operate a parking barrier/entry system
- vehicle access controls should allow disabled people to park before getting out of their vehicle
- the controls should be easy to operate and in an accessible location
- a waiting zone should be provided for those people who may experience difficulty operating an entry (intercom) system.

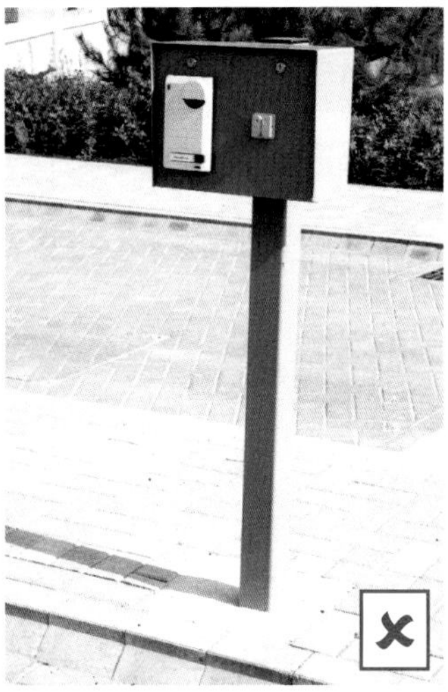

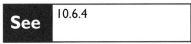

4. To operate this car park control the user needs to be able to:
   - speak
   - hear
   - reach out of the car

   and to

   - have a right arm (in the UK or a left arm in the rest of Europe)
   - have sufficient visual acuity to read the information on the sign.

It is possible to hold a driving licence without any of the above, but you would not be able to gain entry to this car park – simply because of the way it is being managed.

8.5.2 Entry barriers

Proximity sensor or attendant controlled gates and barriers are preferable where feasible, as ticket, swipe card or key activated controls require manual dexterity and upper limb function which may be difficult for some disabled people.

8.5.3 Location of ticket machines

If disabled people are required to purchase car parking tickets, then it is recommended that the ticket machines are located next to the disabled parking bays.

See 10.6.4

8.5.4 Operation of controls

Accessible ticket machines should conform to guidance in BS EN 12414.

For useability, ticket machines should:

- have controls that are 750 mm – 1200 mm above the ground
- have controls that colour contrast with the surrounding area
- have tactile controls
- have controls with levers, projecting tickets, knobs etc, that do not require fine manual dexterity
- have comprehensive, understandable instructions at an accessible height, and in large print.

Extra time should be provided to allow disabled people to use ticket machines and entry/exit systems. Management procedures should be in place to provide additional assistance, for example the provision of a bell-push with instructions to ring three times if difficulty is experienced in using an entry system, or telephone numbers of whom to contact, clearly displayed for mobile phone users.

8.5.5 Gatekeepers/car parking attendants

Controls that involve operating gates, mechanically controlled barriers or ticket machines, will inevitably cause problems for disabled people. A gatekeeper/car park attendant can assist drivers, by removing barriers to improve accessibility. It is recommended that gatekeepers/car park attendants undergo disability awareness training.

8.5.6 Staff vehicles

Access to the car park can be made accessible for disabled members of staff by providing a radio signal to automatically operate the gates/barrier on entry.

8.6 Paths

8.6.1 Safety and convenience

Paths should be safe, convenient and easy to follow with pedestrian controls that are easy to use.

Paths should:

- be direct, clearly defined and well signposted
- be unobstructed and wide enough for wheelchairs to pass each other (see 8.6.2)
- be free of potential hazards for people with visual impairments, such as overhanging branches, overhead signs, outward opening windows or doors, raised manhole covers or uneven surfaces
- if possible, not crossing roadways on the site (see right)
- not have any obstacles such as barriers, turnstiles, gates or steps that cannot be negotiated by disabled people unless a suitable means for by-passing the obstacle has been provided
- have surfaces that are firm, even and slip-resistant

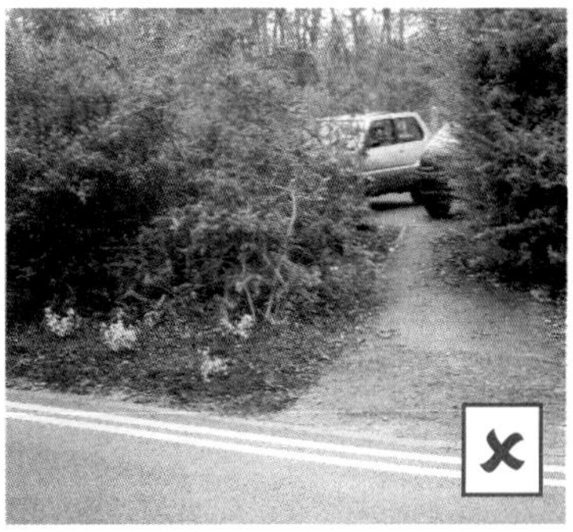

5. Poor on-going management make this really dangerous for everyone.

- be well lit, particularly at changes in surface level
- be provided with resting places not more than 50 m apart and off the main path, for people with mobility impairments.

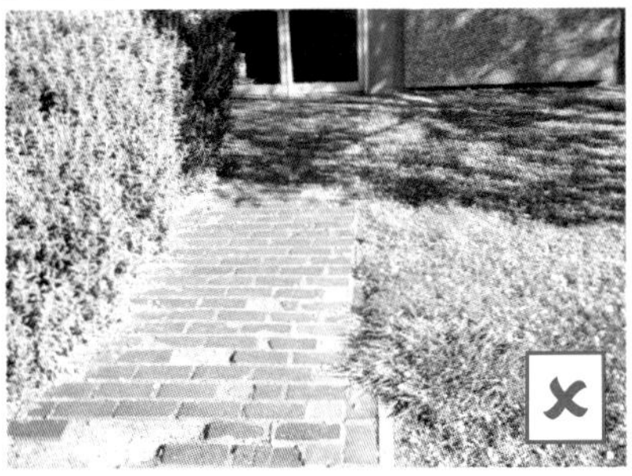

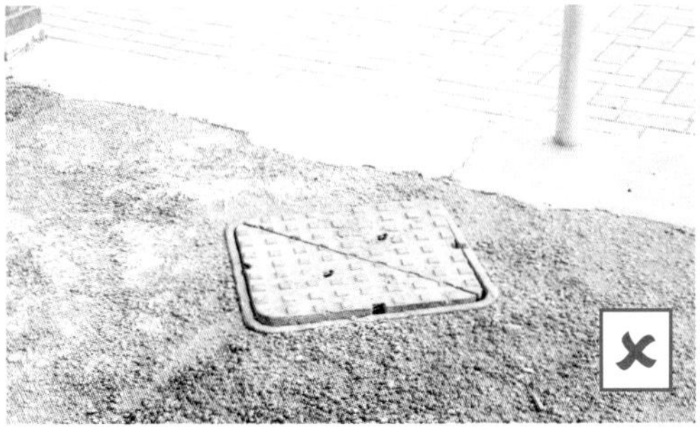

7 & 8. Poorly maintained paths with tripping hazards that are dangerous for all users.

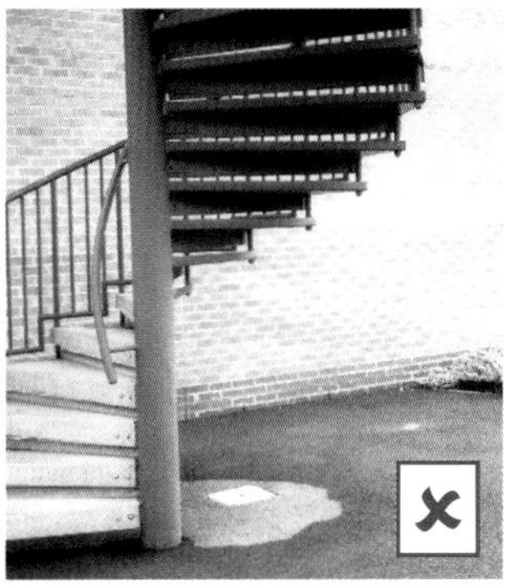

6. A collision accident waiting to happen, especially for someone with poor vision or simply not paying attention.

8.6.2 Detailed design

Dimensions and protection for paths are as follows:

- frequently used paths should be at least 1800 mm wide, which allows for two wheelchair users to pass each other
- a less busy route with passing places should be at least 1500 mm wide and passing places should be 2 m × 1.8 m.

These widths should be maintained up to a height of 2.1 m above ground level as recommended in BS 8300: 2001. (see Figure 8c). A path should be level. Any path with a gradient of more than 1:20 is regarded as a ramp. The cross fall gradient should not exceed 1:50 except when associated with a dropped kerb.

See 9.4

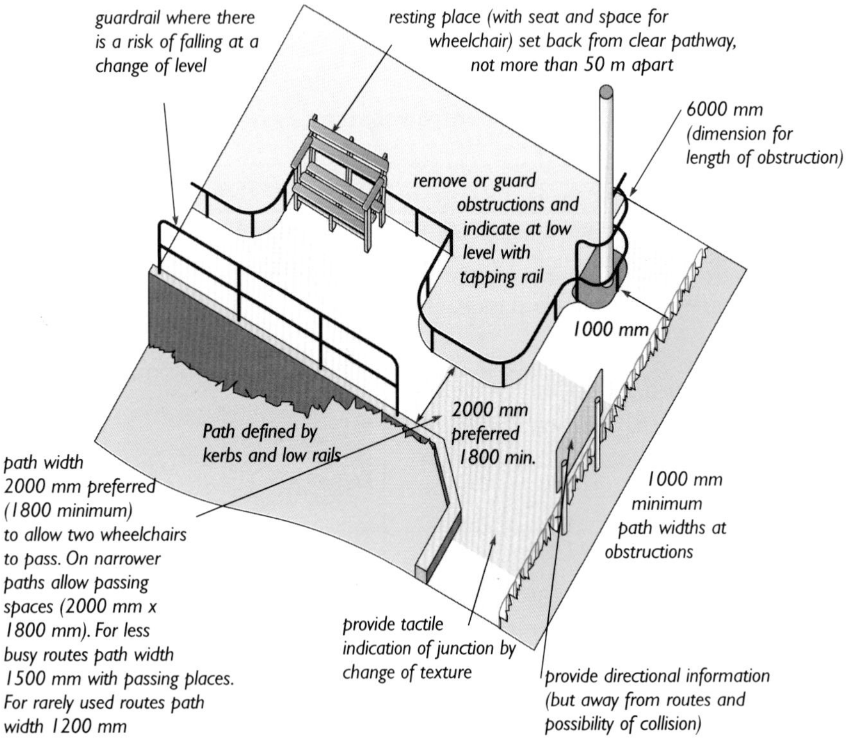

Figure 8c

Dimensions and protection of paths. Defining the edge of the path either with a kerb or a change in texture, for example using grass, will assist orientation and help people with visual impairments. A carefully designed raised kerb could also be used as a tapping rail by people using mobility aids.

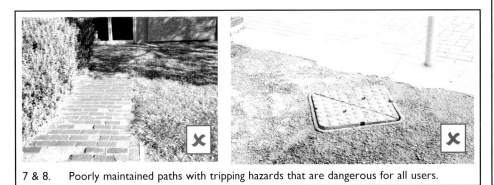

8.6.3 Potential hazards

The location of street furniture is crucial along a pedestrian route as it can present a tripping or collision hazard. It is recommended that litter bins, seats, signposts, bollards and street lights are located at the edge of the route and colour contrasted with the surrounding area.

There are specific guidelines in BS 8300 regarding bollards – they should be at least 1000 mm high and must not be linked by ropes or chains. They should have warning banding at the top of the bollard in a contrasting colour.

Drain covers should not have gaps that exceed 13 mm so that they do not present a tripping hazard for cane users, and should not be positioned in the line of travel.

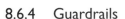

See 8.6.1, 8.6.4

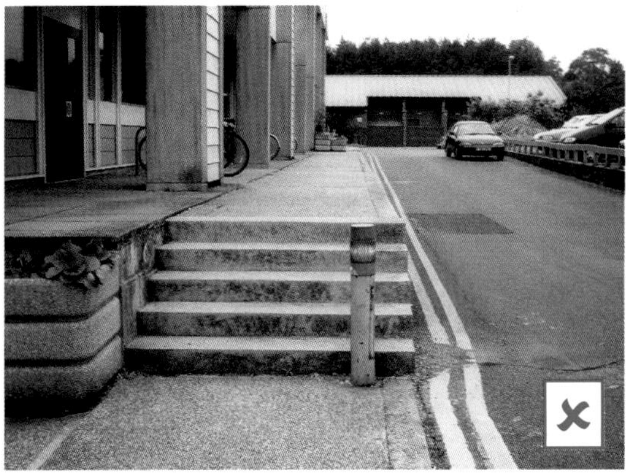

9. Not a well-sited bollard light – and no guardrail or tactile surface is provided to warn of the danger and help prevent people falling over the edge.

8.6.4 Guardrails

Guardrails should be provided if there is a steep drop or slope alongside a path. For safety reasons, wheelchair users and people with visual impairments require guardrails to provide protection from such potential hazards. It is recommended that guardrails should be provided to a height of 1000 mm – 1200 mm above ground level.

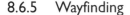

See 8.9.1, 8.9.2

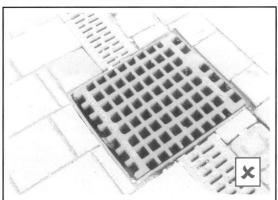

10 & 11 Drainage covers such as these can cause considerable problems for many disabled and non-disabled people.

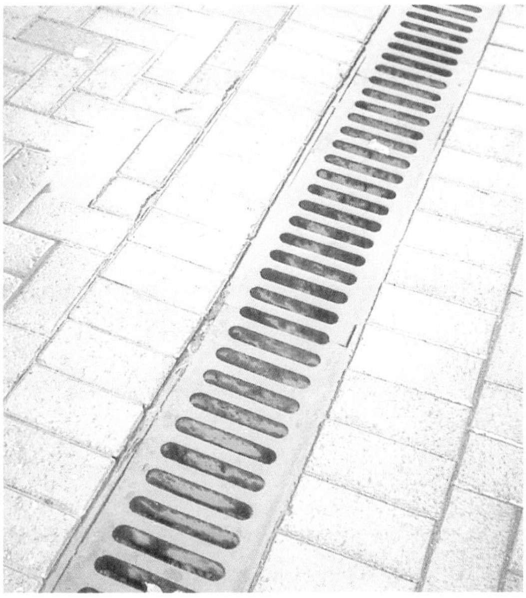

8.6.5 Wayfinding

Wayfinding is the process that all people follow on every journey. There are two main components to the wayfinding process:

- negotiating obstructions or essential features in the environment (such as flights of stairs or road crossings)
- navigating, the process by which people select a route or direction from a number of options.

The whole wayfinding process is dependent upon receiving and processing information. The quicker people are able to do this, and do it accurately, the more rapidly will they complete their journey.

It is possible to assist people with visual impairments to identify and remember a certain route by providing tactile and sensory clues such as changes in texture, various plants and trees with different shapes, colours and fragrances, as well as water features.

8.6.6 Gates

Gates may be needed on paths in certain environments to prevent animals straying, or to restrict access by bicycles or motorbikes. Designers have considered this dilemma and developed gates that can overcome restricting certain users and allowing access for others. The correct design of gates to be installed must be given careful consideration and must not present a barrier to disabled people.

See 8.5.2, 8.5.5, 8.5.6

8.6.7 Narrow paths

Modification of existing paths to make them suitable for use by disabled people may involve changes in dimensions and appearance that are not easily acceptable, particularly where there are historic buildings or monuments. For example, between existing buildings or trees, instead of a 1800 mm wide path allowing wheelchairs to pass easily, a narrower path (a minimum of 1000 mm) could be acceptable as long as it does not extend for more than 6 m and provided there are wider passing places at intervals along the route.

8.6.8 Modifying surfaces

Surfaces present the greatest challenge. Even slightly irregular surfaces will impede wheelchair users and present trip hazards for people with mobility impairments. Surfaces such as cobbles, gravel, muddy patches and grass are very difficult to negotiate for some disabled people and for parents pushing prams, and should be avoided wherever possible. However, it is costly to replace a large surface area which may be an important aesthetic feature of the building.

Laying a 1000 mm wide strip of smooth flags within a cobbled or loose surfaced area, or across or around an area with an uneven surface, is a solution to providing an accessible, well defined route while retaining most of the original surface. Consideration must be given to consulting conservation authorities for listed buildings and monuments.

8.7 Carriageway crossings

8.7.1 Safety and convenience

Crossings should be identifiable, safe and conveniently located for disabled people to use. They should:

- be direct, clearly defined and clearly signposted
- be clearly visible to drivers
- have level crossings and dropped kerbs suitable for unaccompanied wheelchair users
- have appropriate blister tactile surfaces on the path or pavement at each side to alert people with visual impairments that they are approaching a carriageway. The tactile surface should colour contrast with the surrounding area. It is essential that red tactile paving is used only at controlled crossings.

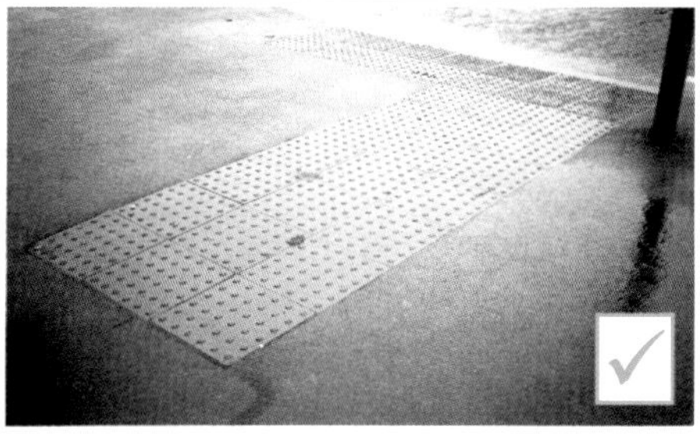

12 & 13 Red coloured paving (above) should be used at controlled crossings only. At uncontrolled crossings buff coloured paving (below) should be used.

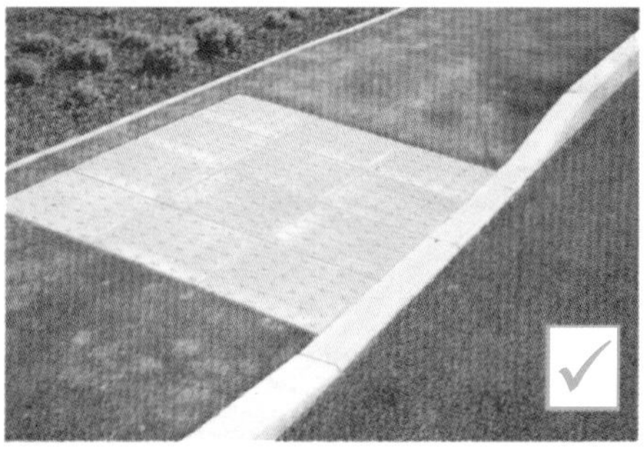

- if there are controlled crossings, ie with traffic lights, audible and visual signals must be provided to give information about when it is safe to cross the road. A rotating cone (a small cone projecting from the underside of the control unit), should be used to give tactile information of when it is safe to cross the road.
- be well lit (see Chapter 13).

8.7.2 Location of crossings

Crossings at street corners are preferred because they are less likely to be obstructed by parked vehicles. It is recommended that the crossing is positioned a short way down the side road where it will be away from the direct line of traffic and the extent of tactile paving will be minimal. Dropped kerbs should not be located on the apex of a corner. To avoid traffic accidents, a crossing between corners needs to be particularly well lit and well marked. The local authority highways department should be consulted over the location of crossings and referral can be made to the Department for Transport's guidance document LTN 1/95.

8.7.3 Design of crossings

The design and details of crossings in different situations are shown in the Department for Transport guidance document LTN 2/95. Level or flush access is essential at crossings. This can be achieved by providing dropped kerbs, or by raising the road level at the crossing itself.

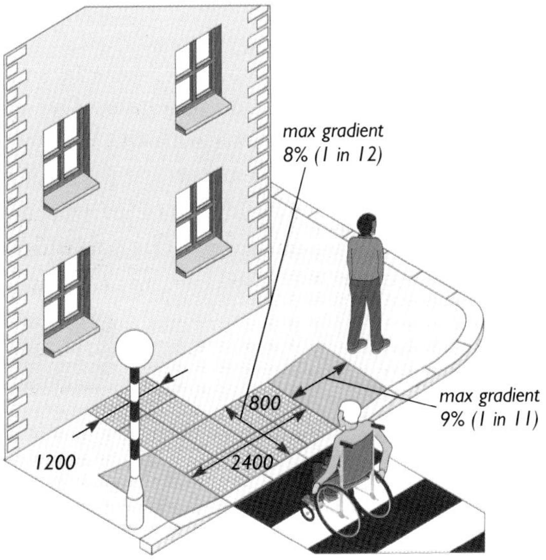

Figure 8d Dropped kerbs should be flush with the road (a maximum 6 mm rounded bull nose edge is the maximum recommended change in level). They should have a maximum gradient of 1:12 on the direct approach and 1:11 on the flared sides. The recommended width of the flush area is the same width as the crossing itself (2400 mm).

8.7.4 Crossings on public highways

Dropped kerbs can be requested on public highways where wheelchair users or people with mobility impairments need to cross or where parking bays and setting down points for disabled people are to be provided.

See 8.2.3

8.7.5 Historic buildings

The modified blister tactile surface recommended by the Department for Transport is the only surface that provides adequate tactile warning of a dropped kerb or crossing. This surface is available in a variety of materials and colours and can be used sensitively within conservation areas.

8.8 Slopes

8.8.1 Accessible slopes

Wheelchair users and other people with restricted mobility should be able to negotiate slopes with ease. Slopes should be gentle and provide regular, level resting places with seats.

8.8.2 Gradients and lengths

Access to a building via a long slope or ramp should be avoided wherever possible. Any slope with a gradient steeper than 1:20 should be regarded as a ramp and supported by handrails and level landings. Cross falls or cambers on slopes can be extremely difficult to negotiate in a wheelchair and should not exceed 1:50.

See 8.1.2, 9.4

8.8.3 Resting places

There should be resting places with seats at least at 50 m intervals along routes. The seats should be placed adjacent to the pedestrian route and should colour contrast with the surrounding area. The seats should be 450 mm – 500 mm high, with a back and with arm rests, preferably on both sides of each seating position. Some seating without arm rests should also be provided. There should be an appropriately sized space next to the seat for a wheelchair. The ground surface to the space must be suitable for use in wet and dry weather conditions.

See 9.4.2

8.8.4 Existing steeper slopes

Many buildings are located on sites or fronting onto pavements that slope at more than 1:12 and are not negotiable by wheelchair users without assistance or by some people with mobility impairments. It is not always possible to solve this problem because of conservation issues, structural constraints or cost implications. However, there are environments where a parking space can be provided at the entrance giving independent access to a disabled person with a car. Alternatively a different entrance could be considered if an equal right to access is provided.

8.9 Handrails and guardrails

8.9.1 Handrails

Handrails should:

- be provided continuously on both sides of slopes or centrally when the unobstructed width exceeds 1800 mm
- be provided between 900 mm and 1000 mm tall and extend 300 mm beyond the top and bottom of the slope
- have positive ends (return back to the wall or down to the floor)

- have surfaces which are smooth, not hot or cold to the touch, and colour contrast with the surrounding area
- have a diameter of 40 mm – 50 mm if circular or, if oval, 50 mm wide × 38 mm deep
- have a clearance of 50 mm – 60 mm wide between the handrail and any adjacent wall.

8.9.2 Guardrails

Guardrails are needed where they can prevent falls or collisions.

They should be provided:

- at the edge of an upper level
- where there is a risk of falling over an edge or down a slope
- where people might walk into obstructions – open windows or projecting fixtures, for example
- where people might walk into the path of traffic along routes where tactile paving has not been used.

Freestanding guardrails should have a low-level rail or be positioned over a raised kerb. This will warn people with visual impairments, who are using a long cane as a mobility aid, of a potential trip hazard. Guardrails should colour contrast with the surrounding area and be turned down to the ground or have a broad, blunt end which does not present a tripping or collision hazard.

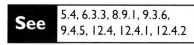

See 5.4, 6.3.3, 8.9.1, 9.3.6, 9.4.5, 12.4, 12.4.1, 12.4.2

8.10 External lighting

8.10.1 Good external lighting

Routes will be easier to follow when:

- there is a uniform general illuminance with increased lighting at changes in level and to illuminate signs
- glare and cross shadows are avoided
- light sources are positioned at spacings which produce a good uniform disribution of light across a space and along a route
- light sources are positioned so that people are not walking in their own shadow. This is particularly important at changes of level.

The safety and security of all people, both actual and perceived, can be increased with good external lighting.

9 Entrances

The entrance into a building is seen by many owners, designers and managers to epitomise how the accessibility of the environment will be viewed. In reality, it is only part of the overall standard by which a building will be judged. However, if access into the environment is not available on an appropriate and equal basis, good design and management within the environment will have reduced value. This chapter discusses the main issues to be considered in providing and managing inclusive, accessible entrances.

See 8.1.3

9.1 Design principles

9.1.1 Independent access

All users should have independent access into the building. People should generally be able to arrive at the most suitable part of the building for the purpose of their visit. Whenever possible, entrances should be provided that allow disabled people to use them without assistance. Entrance arrangements that require assistance from companions or a member of staff should be avoided, but may be the only solution in some existing buildings.

9.1.2 Access principal entrance

Disabled people should not have to use a different entrance from non-disabled people, unless no other solution can be identified or constructed that will allow everyone to share the same entrance. Making disabled people use a special entrance may well be seen as discriminatory, especially if this secondary entrance is of a lower standard than that used by non-disabled people. Entrances that are designated for a particular user group, for example, entrances for staff, students, visitors or ticket holders, should be accessible to both disabled and non-disabled people.

9.1.3 Identifying entrances

All entrances should be signposted clearly and consistently with signs that meet good sign design guidance criteria, for example, upper and lower case lettering in a sans serif font that has good colour contrast and is tactile where appropriate. Identifying accessible entrances assists all users, but especially disabled users.

9.1.4 Visibility of entrances

Entrances should be clearly visible and the use of colour can make doors easier to distinguish when viewed against the façade of the building. If an entrance is fully glazed, the use of manifestation at two heights (within a zone of 1400 mm – 1600 mm from the floor) is essential for safety and visibility for people who are either seated or standing, and for children. Manifestation should contrast in colour and luminance with the background beyond the glazed doors, ie the background against which it is viewed, in all conditions of lighting and use.

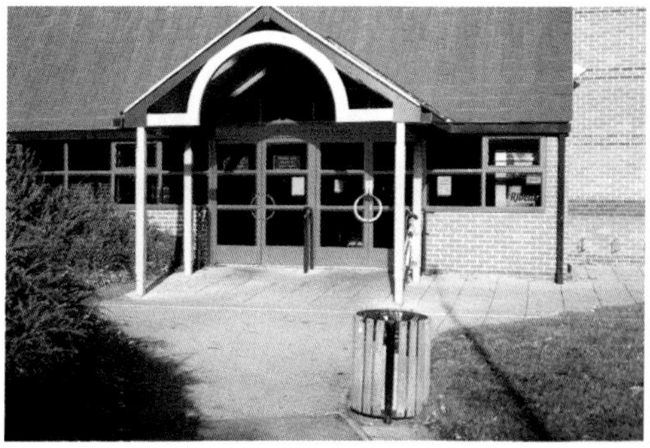

1. The entrance is not well-signed and the door contrast is poor, but the location of the entrance is clearly identified by the design and colouring of the porch.

9.1.5 Provision of shelter

Shelter at entrances is particularly important for disabled people whose movement restrictions, equipment, or sensory impairments, may delay their entry into the building.

9.2 Strategy for existing buildings

9.2.1 Accessible entry

Overcoming inaccessible features to enable entry into an existing building is, in many cases, the key improvement issue. Steps and thresholds, heavy external doors, narrow door leaves and the absence of handrails, are typical of the existing building stock. The entry to most buildings present some obstacle to wheelchair users, or those with mobility impairments. The features that make the entrance inaccessible are often there for traditional or constructional reasons and may also be important to the appearance of the building – particularly in historic buildings. It is not always a straightforward matter to make an entrance accessible. Entry improvements may be the subject of planning or building regulations, as well as requiring permission from the building owner.

9.2.2 Steps at entrances

Steps at the entrance to a building are a barrier to independent access for wheelchair users and some people with mobility impairments. Entrances can be made accessible by:

Landscaping or re-aligning the external surface

This is usually possible only if there are just one or two existing steps at an entrance. Removing the step or steps is often a better solution than providing a ramp, which tends to be more obvious and requires additional manoeuvring space.

Providing a ramp

When there is a flight of more than four or five steps, a ramp will be a very prominent feature. The maximum gradient for a ramp of this height, which, if designed to the guidance in BS 8300: 2001, is likely to be 1:15 (depending on the height of the steps). A ramp will also require a reasonable amount of space which may not be readily available in an existing building.

Installing an external platform lift

This provision may save space, but can usually accommodate only one wheelchair at a time. It requires instructions if the user is not familiar with its operation and may be subject to vandalism. It will also require regular planned maintenance to ensure it is operational when required. However, it is sometimes the only way to provide satisfactory access into a building.

Using a temporary ramp

Temporary or portable ramps should not be used in new buildings. Where it is not possible to provide a fixed permanent ramp in an existing building, a temporary ramp may be seen as a reasonable solution in certain difficult situations, providing it is well managed. However, it should be considered only in those circumstances where more permanent solutions are not practicable or reasonable.

9.2.3 Alternative means of access

Although ramps, platform lifts and raised pavement levels are regularly used to make entrances accessible, the problems associated with improving accessibility at the principal entrance are not always solved by permanent building work. This may be through budget restrictions, existing conservation issues or for practical reasons.

Other alternatives should be considered, such as:

- a new main entrance – developing another entrance (which requires less extensive work or has better access to car parking) into the principal entrance and making the necessary adjustments to the use of the space and to the circulation routes inside the building
- using an alternative entrance which offers entry to the building on an equal basis. An alternative entrance must not represent a lesser standard of facility to that offered to non-disabled people entering and exiting the building.
- an internal link – connecting the building, by an accessible internal route, to an adjacent building where the principal entrance is accessible as long as the route is not excessively or unreasonably long for disabled people to use
- assisted entry – if no entrance can be made accessible, not just in terms of cost but also in terms of what would be considered reasonable in all the circumstances of an individual case under the DDA 1995 (see also Chapter 3), a management policy of providing assisted entry may be acceptable. However, any system that requires users to call for assistance must be accompanied by the appropriate management procedures, which are critical if a user needs help. They must meet the needs of disabled people, and ensure that neither they, nor the staff facilitating assisted entry, are at risk of injury (see also Chapter 4).

Providing a new entrance to be used exclusively by disabled people is not an acceptable solution.

9.2.4 Historic buildings

Chapters 3 and 6 explain the principles on which proposed improvements to historic buildings are judged when listed building applications are considered. Chapter 3 also summarises the planning policy guidelines for considering accessibility in planning applications.

9.2.5 Consultation

Creating an accessible entrance may involve extensive consultation with the local authority, the landlord, tenant, access officer and other relevant bodies. When the principal entrance is to be relocated, or the external appearance of the building radically altered, people will need to be advised that the changes are necessary. It is always advisable to enlist the support of local access groups and disabled people who would use the accessible entrance. Attitudes to accessibility are changing with the influence of the DDA, and people have a greater awareness of the reasoning behind such changes.

9.2.6 Other improvements

Inaccessible entrances should not prevent the implementation of other improvements within a building. Many features such as suitable signage, information in alternative formats, the use of colour contrast and the provision of auxiliary aids, can be introduced to provide an accessible environment for all users.

9.3 External Steps

9.3.1 Accessible step requirements

Accessible steps should:

Visibility

- be appropriately lit.

Ease of approach

- be covered, where possible, so the user is protected from the weather
- have a minimum clear width of the stepped access route of 1000 mm
- avoid single steps wherever possible
- have individual flights of not more than 12 risers.

Usability

- have appropriately designed handrails, provided in materials which take into account the needs of disabled people.

Good communication

- have a corduroy tactile surface at the top and bottom of external steps, where possible
- have contrasting nosings to help people with sensory impairments
- have handrails which are contrasted in terms of colour and luminance with the supporting wall or the background against which they will be viewed.

Safety of use

- have slip resistant surfaces, especially when wet
- have a shallow pitch, a generous tread width and landings not too far apart so they are easier to negotiate
- always be provided as an alternative to ramps
- have a handrail provided on both sides of the steps for use with either hand.

See 11.5.2

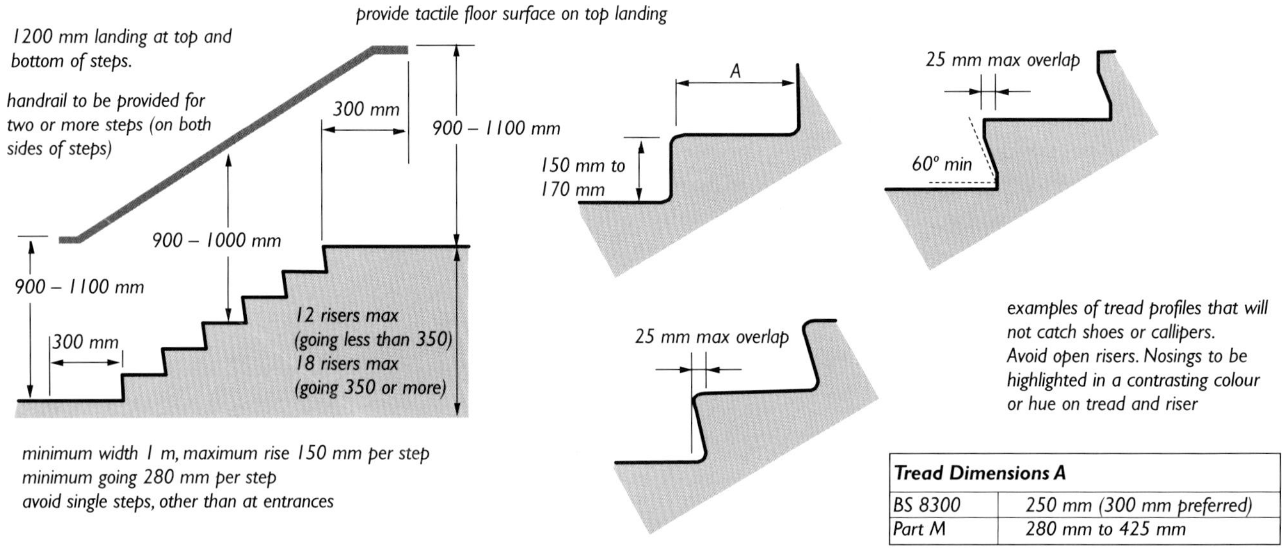

Tread Dimensions A	
BS 8300	*250 mm (300 mm preferred)*
Part M	*280 mm to 425 mm*

Figure 9a Recommendations for external steps

9.3.2 Dimensions

The recommended guidelines for external steps and stairs are summarised in Figure 9a.

9.3.3 Design details

The profile of the tread or riser, the surface finish of the steps and landings and the detail of handrails are critical for people with sensory or mobility impairments. Open risers, deeply recessed risers and projected nosings should not be used because they can catch toes of shoes or callipers. Treads should be slip-resistant and have contrasting nosings that are visible when both ascending and descending the stairs.

Landings at the top and bottom of external steps should have a corduroy tactile surface to alert people with sensory impairments that they are approaching a stair. Care must be taken to ensure that the coefficient of friction of the material forming the tactile surface is similar to that of the surrounding surface. If not, a serious stumbling hazard may be created.

9.3.4 Steps from the pavement

Where a building has a step up from the pavement or footpath, there may be several ways to address or overcome the physical obstacle, each one depending upon the particular circumstances of the original layout. These options include:

- **Changing the position of the opening**. This option may be available if the pavement slopes along the face or side of the building.
- **Lowering a section of the floor inside the building**. This may provide space for an internal ramp.
- **Recessing the entrance to provide an external porch**. This may provide sufficient space for an external ramp. Consideration may be given to either recessing the door or, if possible, part of the façade. This also offers the additional advantage of providing shelter but may, at the same time, reduce valuable (not just in terms of cost) usable floor space inside the building.
- **Realigning the pavement or landscaping**. It is better to change the level of pavement outside the building to address the obstacle, rather than try to remodel the building.

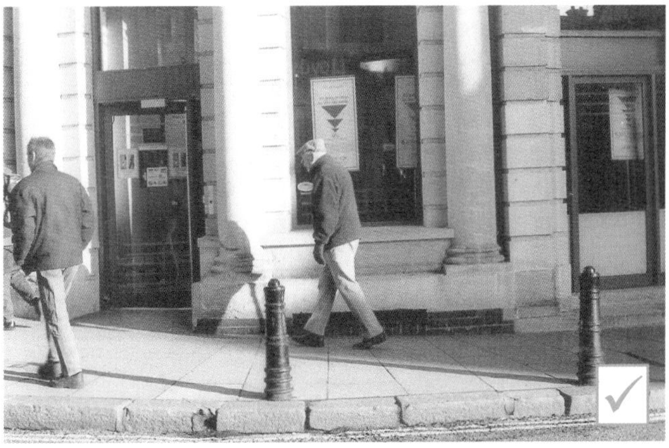

2. The original entrance was on the right. Moving the entrance to the new position took advantage of the sloping pavement to provide a level entrance

9.3.5 Realigning pavements and landscaping

Raising a pavement or path is generally easier than lowering it, where, for example, services may be affected by excavation works. Also, realignment may address the needs of several properties, making it more cost effective. If historic buildings are involved, care must be taken to avoid obscuring important details such as plinths, column bases and archaeological evidence. Clearly, if this is a possibility, permission will need to be sought from relevant authorities.

Other factors that may need to be considered include the location of other entrances and the width of pavements. Consultation with, and the approval of, relevant authorities may be required.

9.3.6 Handrails

Handrails should be provided on both sides of steps and must always be provided, even for a single step. The provision of an additional central handrail on wider flights offers better access to a handrail when there are many people using the steps.

Handrails on both sides are essential to assist:

- assistance dog users, who cannot use a handrail if it is provided only on the side of the assistance guide dog
- people with visual impairments who
- use a long cane for mobility
- people who have paralysis to one side of their body
- people carrying items.

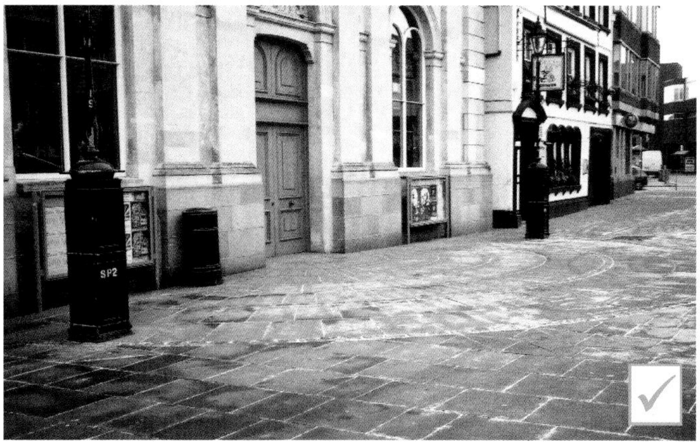

3. An excellent example of how external work to realign the pavement has overcome the step into this historic building. The design of the pavement has also been used as subtle indicator of the location of the entrance.

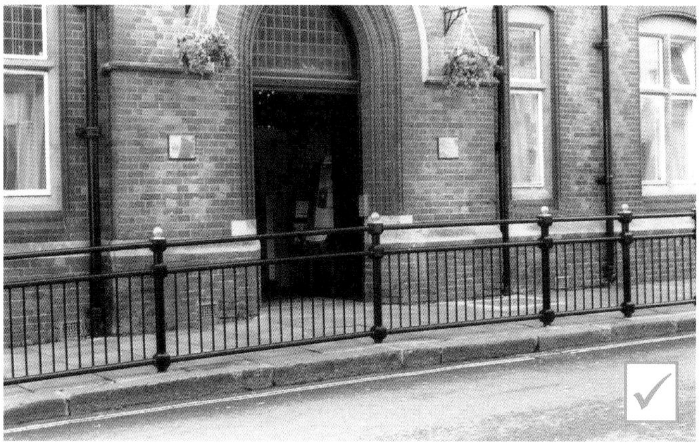

4. A further good example of the ability to overcome a step into the building with careful pavement realignment. See Chapter 7 Case studies (Newbury Town Hall).

The recommended dimensions for handrails are 40 mm – 50 mm if circular in design and 38 mm × 50 mm if oval. Handrails should extend 300 mm horizontally beyond the top and bottom of the steps, and have positive ends. The horizontal extension allows for a person to gain information about the presence of a stair, when it begins to ascend or descend, and to gain support before using the stairs. The positive end assists in reducing the risk of clothing being caught as the handrail is approached.

Handrails should contrast in terms of colour and luminance with the surrounding area and be continuous around all landings and half landings. It is good practice to provide surface coatings on handrails that are warm to the touch.

Handrails should take into account the needs of children or people of short stature when using the steps. The provision of handrails at two heights is strongly recommended.

9.4 Ramps

If a flight of steps is all that is visible at the principal entrance to a building, people who need to use a ramp may not search for a concealed ramp and simply avoid the building. In most circumstances, directional signage could be used, but it is no substitute for being able to see that the building is accessible, something which adds to a feeling of being welcomed rather than excluded. However, in some situations, a ramp, which presents an imposing object if it has several slopes and landings, may be visually intrusive at the entrance to a building of historical or architectural interest. If this is so, some concealment or blending in of the ramp may be justifiable, but such action should always be the exception rather than the rule.

Concealment or blending in for architectural or historical reasons must never compromise equal accessibility for all.

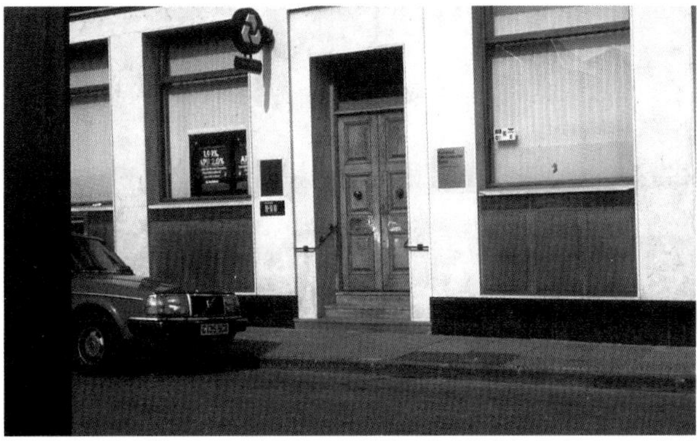

5. The original entrance to this largely inaccessible public access building.

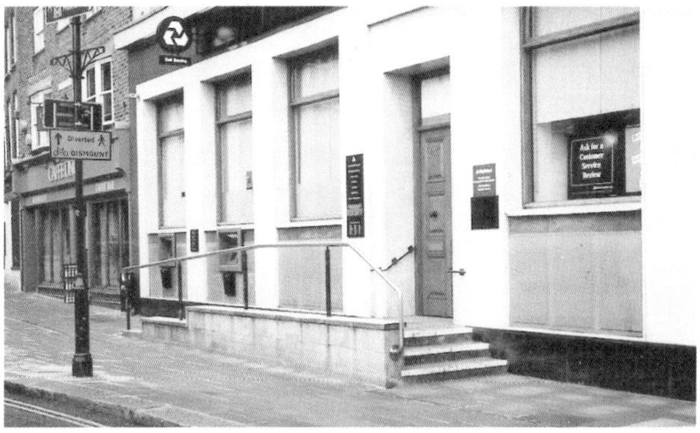

6. Alterations to the external pavement area allowed the provision of a ramped and stepped entrance, which has improved access for everyone.

If steps are provided, ramps should be provided as an alternative route. They must never be used to replace steps, as some disabled people find ramps difficult to use and prefer to use steps.

A ramp can also fulfil many other functions and should not be considered as being exclusively for the use of disabled people. It can be a valuable access aid for people pushing prams, carrying luggage, or making deliveries. However, none of these activities should be carried out in a way that prevents or restricts disabled people using the ramp when required.

See 6.3.3, 9.2.2, 9.4.1, 9.4.3, 9.4.5, 9.4.6, 9.4.7, 11.6

9.4.1 Accessible ramps

The main design consideration must always be that ramps should be considered only where it is necessary to overcome unavoidable changes in level.

In an existing situation a ramp may need to be introduced to overcome changes in level. However, in a new design or major refurbishment, ramps should never be used simply to overcome steps or changes of level that have been introduced, but could have been avoided.

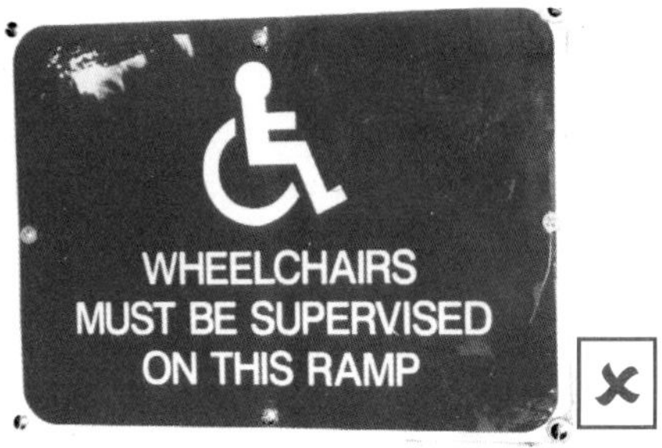

7. Not an inclusive message to users of the buildings. Why does someone need "supervision" and how do they get it?

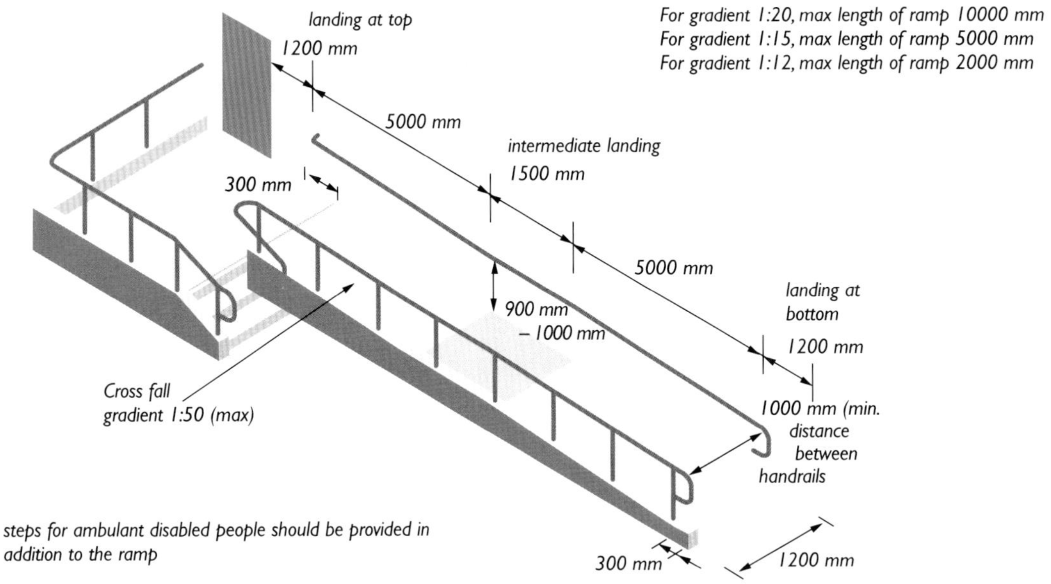

Figure 9b Requirements for ramps

Design considerations

Generally:

- ramps should be suitable for independent access by wheelchair users. Their design should conform to the guidance given in Figure 9b
- steps should always be provided as an alternative if a ramp has a gradient of 1:20 or steeper
- to minimise the effect of tiredness, no section of a ramp should exceed 10 m in length or 500 mm in rise
- a gradient of 1:15 is acceptable, but 1:12 is the absolute maximum. A gradient of 1:12, whilst being the maximum, will still be too steep for some disabled people to use and may prevent them accessing a building.
- the minimum surface width should be 1200 mm
- ramps less than 1800 mm wide will not allow two wheelchair users to pass each other. If it is not possible to see the whole of the ramp from top to bottom before starting to use it, the surface width of the ramp must exceed 1800 mm. If this is not possible, passing places must be provided
- ramps of the minimum width of 1200 mm should not exceed 5 m in length.

9.4.2 Landings

Level landings along a ramp can be used as resting places (1500 mm by the width of the ramp) or passing places if they are large enough (min 1800 mm × 1800 mm).

A level landing (1200 mm by the width of the ramp) should also be provided at the top and bottom of a ramp and at changes in direction. This will assist wheelchair users in manoeuvring onto and off the ramp, or between sections. If a ramp is not under cover, the surface should be provided with a cross fall not exceeding 1:50, and appropriate drainage holes in upstands to dispel surface water.

See 9.4.4

9.4.3 Surfaces

The surface of a ramp should be of a slip-resistant material (even when wet), and should be firm, and easy to clean and maintain.

Where different materials are used for the ramp, landings and approaches to it, it is important that the coefficients of friction of the material used are similar. This will minimise the risk of stumbling.

A tactile surface (corduroy pattern) to alert people with visual impairments must not be used at the top or bottom of ramps. This surface is intended for use at steps and stairs only and may cause confusion and potential danger if incorrectly used.

See 9.3.3

9.4.4 Upstands

To protect against falling, and to act as a "tapping rail" for visually impaired people who are long cane users, an upstand or barrier at least 100 mm high should be provided for the full length of the ramp and landings. The upstand should also contrast in terms of colour and luminance with surroundings. Further guidance is also given in BS 6180.

9.4.5 Handrails to ramps

Handrails should be provided on both sides of a ramp for ramps longer than 2 m. For ramps less than 2 m, a handrail can be provided on one side only, but both sides are preferred. This will assist ambulant disabled people or those who, being weaker on one side of their body, may benefit from additional physical support when ascending or descending a ramp – whatever its length. People with visual impairments will also use handrails on ramps for tactile information.

Generally:

- the minimum clear distance between handrails should be 1000 mm
- the top edge of the handrail should be between 900 mm and 1000 mm above the surface level of the ramp and landings
- the design of the handrail should extend 300 mm beyond the top and bottom of the ramp and be continuous along or around landings. Any extension should not present an obstruction to the safe and easy use of the ramp.

For guidance on the design of handrails, see Figure 9a.

9.4.6 Lighting to ramps

Artificial lighting at the top, bottom and along the whole length of the ramp should be evenly distributed with an illuminance of at least 100 lux.

For general guidance on the design of lighting see Chapter 13.

9.4.7 Removable ramps

In some cases, it may be necessary to fit a removable or temporary ramp that is clearly not part of the permanent structure. This may be necessary at the entrance to a building of historical interest where alterations of, or fixings to, the listed facade or steps may not be permitted. Removable ramps often look crude and cumbersome but they can, with care, be designed and constructed to be aesthetically acceptable. Sectional ramps for greater changes in level may, with the handrails, be too bulky to be easily portable. If they are used regularly they need to be solidly constructed and, even though they are portable, may require planning permission. For occasional use, a temporary ramp can be of lighter weight and of less weather resistant construction.

It should always be ensured that appropriate management procedures are in place for the maintenance and storage of removable ramps, and that any health and safety requirements relating to lifting and handling by staff, are addressed.

In some cases, an appropriate solution may involve the positioning of a ramp only when it is needed. This is perhaps easier to arrange in meeting the needs of an employee, but could cause considerable problems if adopted by a service provider. For some buildings, for example those of historical or architectural interest where permission for alterations cannot be gained, this may be seen as all that can reasonably be achieved. Each case will have to be considered on individual circumstances.

Only appropriately trained personnel should provide assistance to disabled people using temporary ramps.

9.5 Entry systems

Where provided, entry systems should be located and designed to allow easy approach and use. Entry systems must be suitable to meet the needs of all users, including those with speech impairments, limited dexterity and visual or hearing impairments.

Entry systems should:

Visibility

- be clearly identifiable (perhaps by using colour and luminance contrast).

Ease of approach

- be located at a maximum 1200 mm above finished floor level (affl).

Usability

- be provided with useable keypads (including the use of embossed numbers and letters).

Communication

- be provided with an induction coupler and an LED display.

Safety of use

- be supported by tested management procedures to offer assistance when requested
- be provided with clear instructions on how to use them.

It may be possible to replace an existing unsatisfactory system with an alternative, perhaps incorporating CCTV. If used, CCTV can greatly enhance the opportunities available to those managing a building or providing services in it.

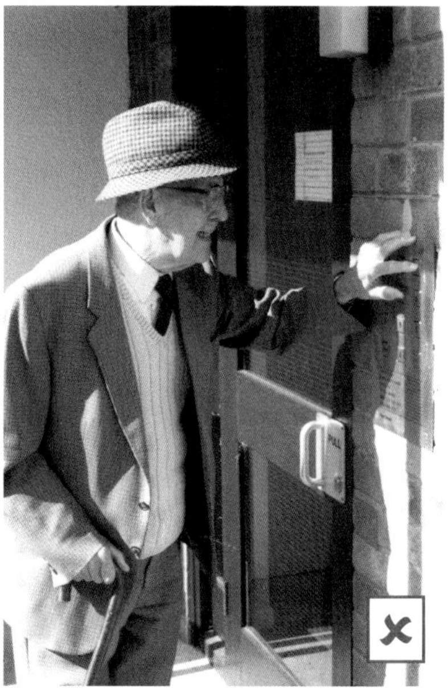

8. Entry control systems can present a stressful, possibly insurmountable, barrier to accessibility if they are not designed to meet the needs of the people who will use them.

Good visual, tactile and audible information is critical, as is the use of appropriate materials.

Unfortunately none of those has been used here.

See 8.5.4

9.6 Door design (except fire exit doors)

9.6.1 Good principles in door design (internal and external doors)

All doors provided within a building should be safe and easy for disabled people to use and should be maintained so that they are always functioning correctly.

Generally, all doors should:

Visibility

- use colour and luminance contrast to identify the door from its background
- be consistent in the location and design of door ironmongery throughout the building.

Ease of approach

- be either automatically operated and opened or require the appropriate force for manual opening
- have adequate space for wheelchair users to manoeuvre, operate and pass through the doorway
- if fully-glazed swing doors, be automatically operated or opened, or fitted with electrically powered hold-open devices which conform to BS EN 1155
- have an unobstructed opening width, not encroached into by door furniture and door stops.

Usability

- use, if fitted, electrically operated push pad controls (rather than electric push button) which are easy to approach and use
- have door closers on swing doors, if fitted, which have adjustable power and conform to BS EN 1154
- be provided with easy-to-use door furniture, preferably lever handles, fingerplates and kicking plates which contrast in colour and luminance with the door
- not be provided with spherical or circular door furniture, for example, door knobs
- use "D-shaped" handles to assist when pulling the door open.

Good communication

- be provided with vision panels that extend down to 500 mm affl.

Safety of use

- be provided with 400 mm deep kick plates to reduce the risk of injury and to protect doors, particularly from damage caused by impact with the footrests of wheelchairs
- if glazed, be provided with manifestation on the glass at two heights for people both seated and standing
- have edges of glass doors highlighted when open (BS 6262 *Guidance on the design of glass doors*).

While many of the good design principles are common to the provision and use of all doors in a building, there are some requirements and recommendations that are specific to where the door is situated. Additional issues specifically related to entrance doors are given here; those specifically related to internal doors are given in 11.4.

9.6.2 Safety and ease of use of entrances, lobbies and external doors

Entrances should:

- be level and provide sufficient level space outside doors for wheelchair users to position themselves
- be wide enough, large enough and positioned appropriately for disabled users to pass through them with ease.

Lobbies should:

- be suitably lit to provide a transition from external to internal lighting
- be wide enough, large enough and positioned appropriately for disabled users to pass through them with ease
- have firm, level floor surfaces to allow wheelchairs to pass over them comfortably
- have appropriate entrance mats provided immediately inside the entrance/lobby.

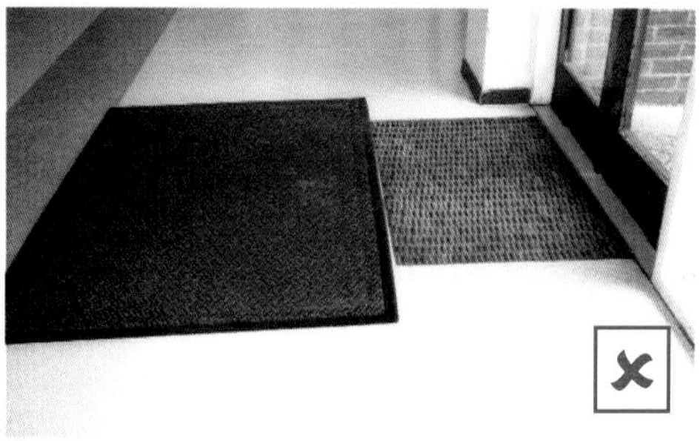

9. The entrance mat is too small, and the use of a loose mat presents a tripping hazard for all users. With floor finishes that are smooth, and potentially slippery when wet, the provision of appropriate entrance mats is critical.

External doors should:

- have handles at the correct height
- have handles that are easy to grip and use
- be opened without involving undue force, risk of collision or risk of being trapped
- have level thresholds, wherever possible.

9.6.3 Automatic doors

Automatically operated and power assisted doors are easier to use by everyone.

There are many types of automatic doors and the benefits of each type can be summarised as follows:

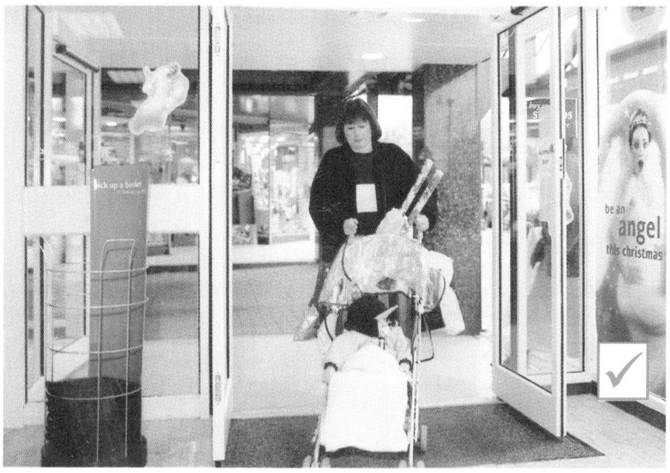

10. Automatic doors can assist everybody.

Sliding doors

- are ideal where the required opening width is available
- are ideal where the area of safety is small and easy to protect
- can be telescopic in operation to enlarge the opening
- can be single or bi-parting
- can be used to increase or maximise the amount of lobby space available
- are useful in areas where there is heavy traffic.

Swing doors

- existing swing doors can be automated
- are the solution if there is a narrow opening with no room at the side

- can assist good directional traffic flow
- can be single or double
- can be appropriate where there is heavy traffic.

Folding doors

- are ideal where fast-acting opening is required
- are good where sliders or swingers cannot be used
- provide an efficient use of space
- can be fitted into existing openings, across corridors and in areas of limited space where other types of automatic door would be difficult to fit
- when used internally do not need a floor mounted track, which assists in providing a level threshold.

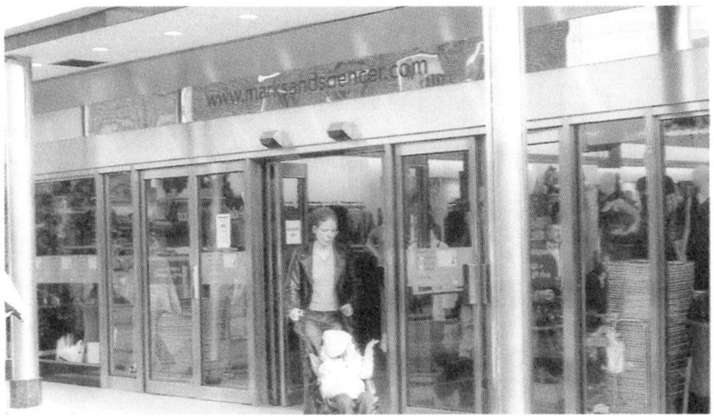

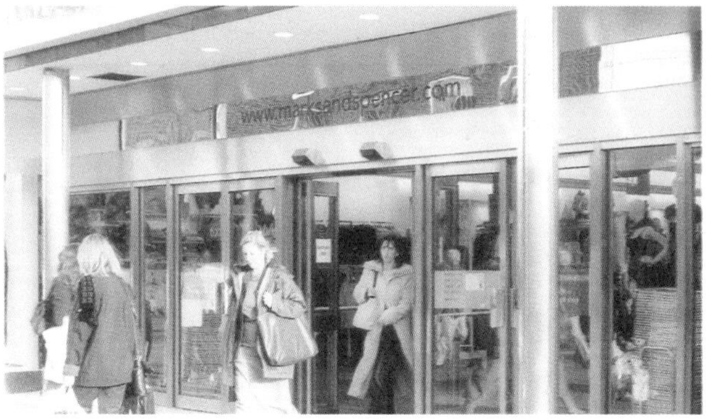

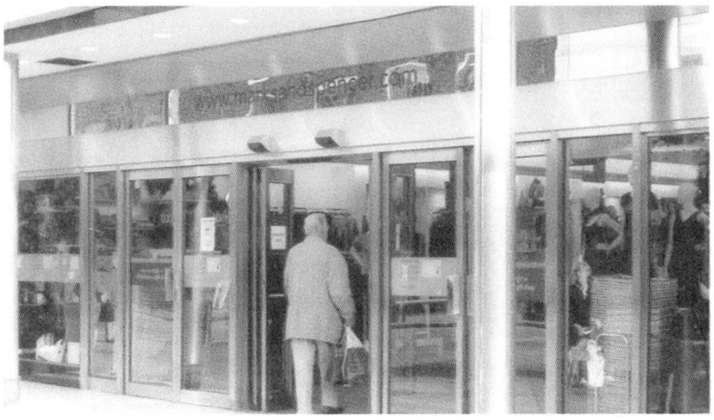

11, 12 & 13.

Given the choice, many people prefer to use automatic, in this case, bi-folding doors.

Low energy/power assisted

- are ideal for internal doors that need to be automated
- have a very low safety risk.

Revolving doors (for further information refer to paragraph 9.6.4)

- are good for preventing draughts
- can offer a good level of security
- can regulate pedestrian flow.

In general, automatic doors should:

- be adjusted to meet the mobility speeds of all users

- have comprehensive fail safe systems, linked to the fire alarm or smoke detection system, that opens (or in some cases) closes doors in the event of a power failure
- be fitted to BS 7036
- have photocell safety sensors that ensure doors cannot open or close if there is an obstruction present
- be provided with side screens that can be removed manually in an emergency
- if swing doors, be fitted with guard rails to protect the door swing area.

Folding doors can be provided with a tactile change of floor surface in front of the door to alert people with a visual impairment about the direction of the door opening.

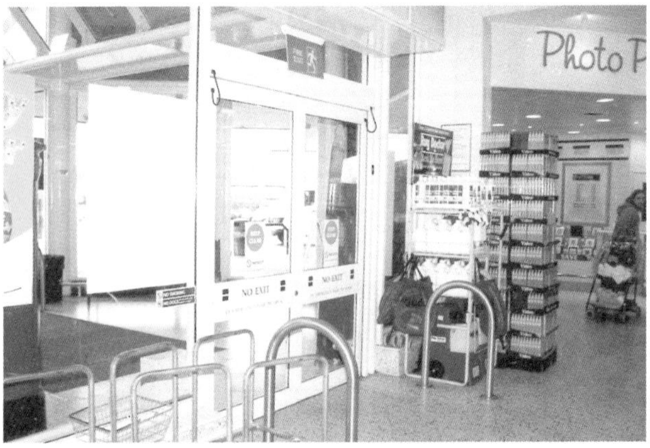

14. An example of guard rails to protect the door swing. Management procedures that allow this amount of clutter clearly need attention.

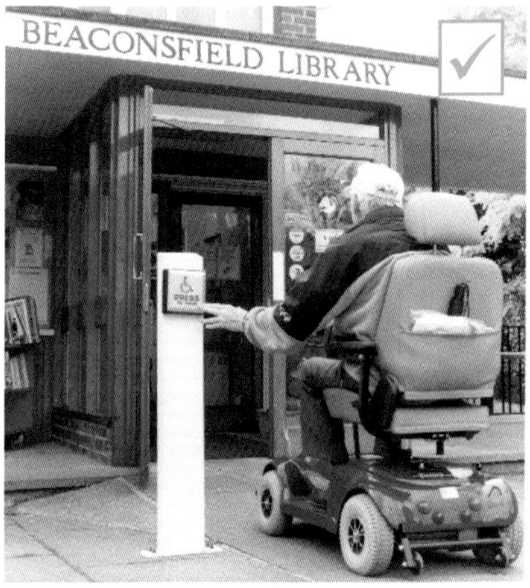

15. A good example of an automatic door that has been adjusted to meet the needs of everyone

9.6.4 Revolving doors

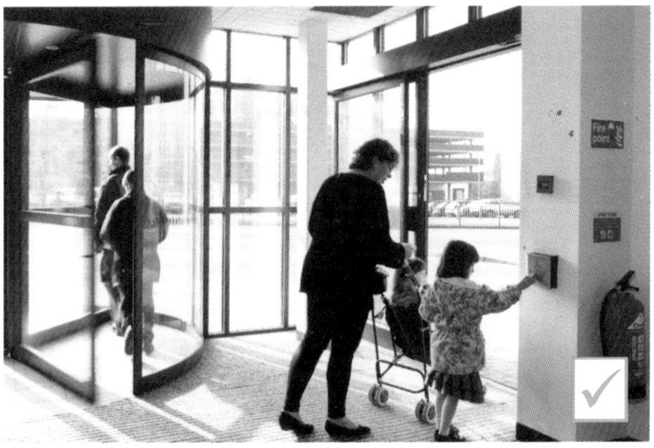

16. There should always be an alternative entrance to a revolving door. This alternative door should have a minimum clear opening width of 800 mm.

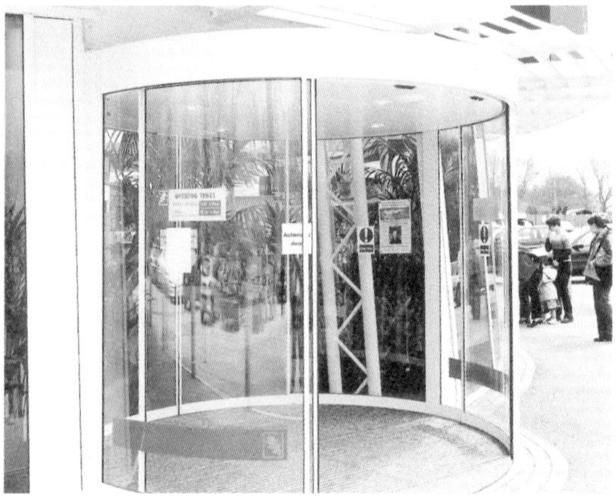

17. Curved sliding doors can provide a good automatic opening, entrance.

Revolving doors do not often provide appropriate access for many disabled people. Larger revolving doors, which are sometimes found in supermarkets or shopping centres, can be more appropriate because more manoeuvring space is available. However, even these larger doors do pose some problems for disabled people. Smaller automatic and manual revolving doors can be stressful to use, particularly for older people and disabled people using mobility aids such as assistance dogs, mobility canes or crutches, which require more manoeuvring space.

In an existing building, if a revolving door is provided, there must be an alternative entrance with a clear opening width of 800 mm immediately adjacent to the revolving door and clearly visible. The door should be automatic, and operational at all times when the revolving door is in use.

Wherever possible, the use of revolving doors in any designs for new work or major refurbishments should be avoided.

9.6.5 Manoeuvring area

It is essential that sufficient manoeuvring space is provided immediately in front of and immediately inside entrance doors. This will allow disabled people to approach the door in a manner that best suits their individual requirements. Management procedures are needed to ensure that items such as goods and luggage are not left standing in the manoeuvring space.

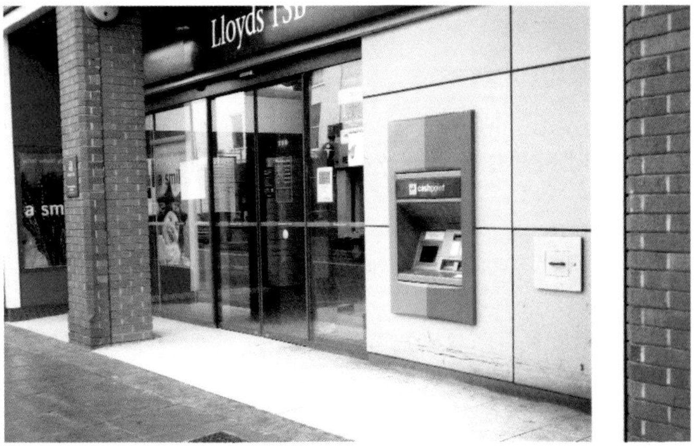

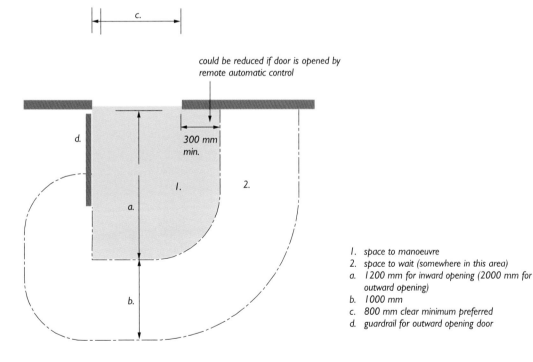

18. Sufficient space is available but the position of the column reduces options for approach. A different design from the entrance, which is likely to have been designed after the position of the column was decided, might have avoided this.

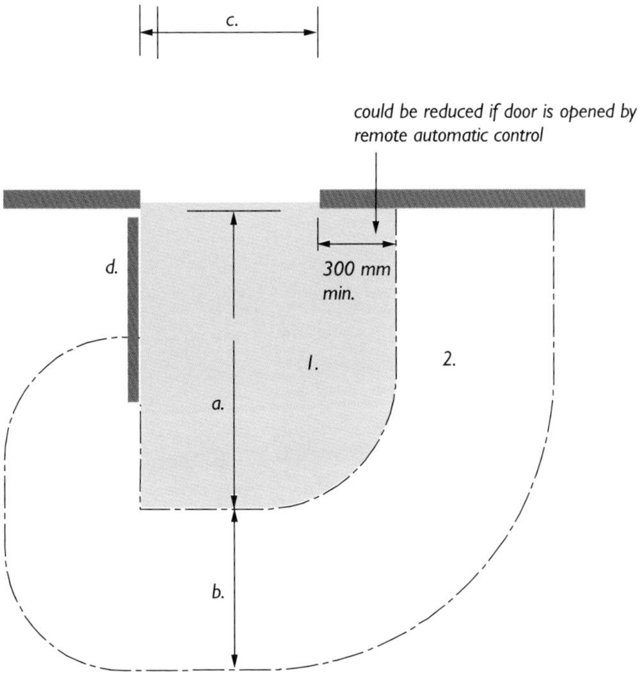

1. *space to manoeuvre*
2. *space to wait (somewhere in this area)*

a. *1200 mm for inward opening (2000 mm for outward opening)*
b. *1000 mm*
c. *800 mm clear minimum preferred*
d. *guardrail for outward opening door*

Figure 9c Space requirements at an entrance

9.6.6 Door widths

The minimum clear opening width for an entrance door is 800 mm, although 900 mm is preferred. Where an entrance is through a lobby, the same minimum width requirement applies to the inner doors.

9.6.7 Entrance mats

Entrance mats should be flush with the floor, fixed, firm and large enough to dry the wheels of a wheelchair. Mat wells should never present a tripping hazard. Coir matting is not suitable for wheeled passage.

See 9.6.2

9.6.8 Door furniture

Door furniture should be distinguishable, in terms of colour and luminance contrast, from the door. It should be easily reached, gripped and operated with minimum effort.

Kicking plates should be securely fixed to the door. If screws are used, they should be countersunk. The material used for the kicking plate must be robust.

See 9.6.1, 16.3.3

9.6.9 Glazing to doors

External and internal doors should not be fully glazed unless they are provided with automatic opening devices. If fully glazed, the glass must be identified with permanent, clearly visible manifestation at a height of between 1400 mm and 1600 mm affl. Manifestation should colour contrast with the background against which it will be viewed, in all artificial and natural lighting conditions. Providing manifestation at two heights, to assist children and people of short stature, is strongly recommended.

Vision panels should give a minimum zone of visibility between 500 mm and 1500 mm affl. Guidance on alternative ways of providing vision panels is given in BS 8300: 2001.

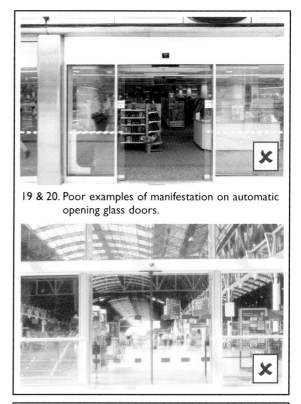

19 & 20. Poor examples of manifestation on automatic opening glass doors.

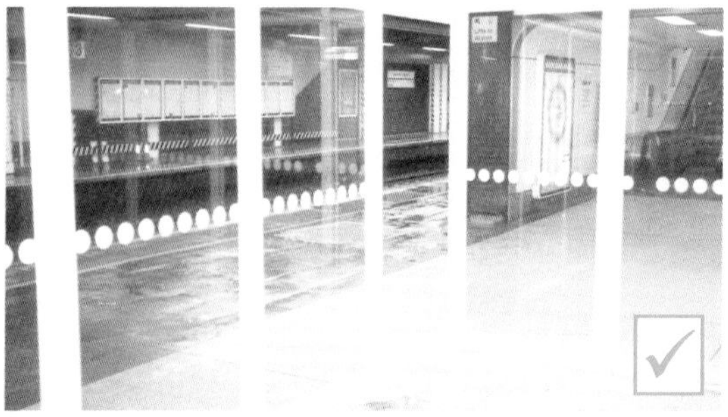

21. Good use of manifestation in terms of contrast but, unfortunately, it is provided at only one height. However, that would be easy to rectify.

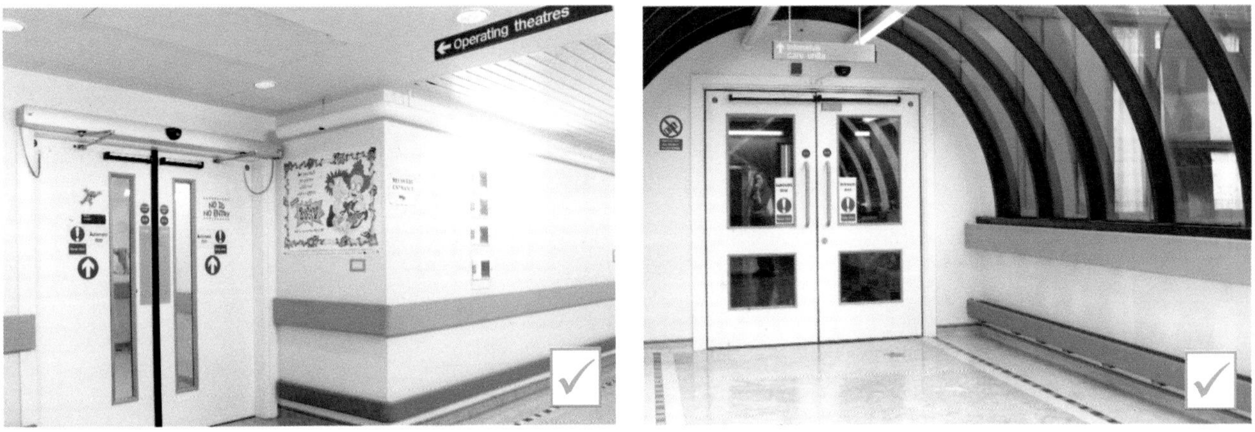

22 &23. These vision panels will help wheelchair users and people with a hearing impairment to see whether anybody is approaching the door from the opposite direction. However, the picture on the left shows how the amount of signage could be very visually confusing.

10 Reception

The importance of the reception area within a building cannot be over-emphasised. For many users it will be the first point at which they can obtain assistance. Importantly, it may also be the first opportunity for providers of services or managers of environments to identify the needs of particular users and move to address them. This represents a point of control at which, with good management practices and staff training, problems that both disabled and non-disabled people may experience when using a building or environment can be identified.

10.1 Design principles

10.1.1 Need for orientation

The first requirement for anyone arriving inside an unfamiliar building is orientation.

Typical concerns that people may have will include:

- Where do I go?
- Who can I ask?
- What am I expected to do?
- Is there a toilet and washroom facility here?
- Where can I sit or wait?
- Can I keep my belongings with me? If not, is there somewhere safe to leave them?
- How do I get out?

For someone with mobility, sensory or cognition impairments, or a learning difficulty, arrival at a building can cause additional problems and stress. They may be asking:

- What are they telling me?
- What do those signs say?
- How do I get to where I want to go?
- Why is the lighting so poor?

10.2 Strategies for existing buildings

10.2.1 Priorities

While there may be several issues to deal with in an arrival space, it is the issues of pedestrian control, manoeuvring space and changes of level that really must be addressed and overcome.

The removal or bypassing of obstacles, such as turnstiles, barriers and changes in level, must be a major consideration. Management procedures should be considered only if changes cannot be made. Prioritisation should be given to the measures that will have the maximum impact on improving accessibility. In complex buildings, this could be clear signage, the provision of accessible reception counters and good, on-going, staff training. In buildings where visitors must wait to be seen or for an event to begin, seating and toilet facilities should be given priority. Areas in which disabled people are required to wait must be warm and draught free, especially when external doors are constantly being opened.

10.2.2 Achievable improvements

Even in major refurbishments, ideal arrival and waiting areas may be difficult to achieve. Lifts and stairs may not be logically placed or there may be columns obstructing the view of reception. Existing structural layouts may also restrict manoeuvring space.

However, it should be generally possible to arrange:

- good lighting
- a decoration scheme that incorporates appropriate colour and luminance contrast
- an acceptable acoustic environment
- floor surfaces that can be negotiated without difficulty.

It is not only disabled users or visitors who would benefit from such attention to detail.

10.3 Easy to use arrangements

Reception areas should:

Visibility

- have a suitably-defined path, using colour and luminance contrast and tactile surfaces from the entrance doors to the counter of the reception desk.

Ease of approach

- have at least one section of desk and counter which is at the correct height and profile for a wheelchair user to use comfortably
- have sufficient clear space in front of the desk and counter for a wheelchair user or someone with an ambulant disability to manoeuvre.

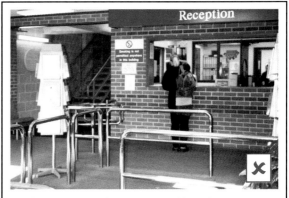

1. This reception desk is very visible with the use of good signage and lighting. The rails clearly define the route to the reception desk. However, there is no lowered section and the turnstile control gate would be impossible for some disabled people to use.

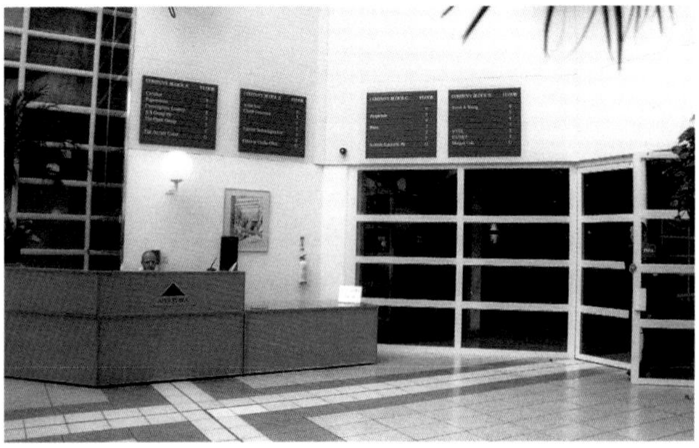

2. Two heights of reception desk have been provided, although there is no knee recess. There is plenty of space in the reception area away from the main entrance door which will avoid congestion. The distinctive floor pattern could give the appearance of steps for people with limited vision.

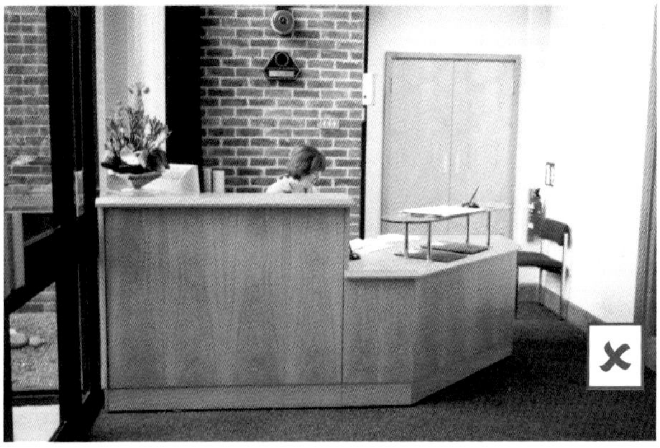

3. The lack of space immediately in front of this reception desk will cause the area to be congested, particularly when several people are using the entrance doors.

Usability

- be of a design which is suitable for use by wheelchair users who are either staff or visitors.

Good communication

- be provided with a sound amplification system (eg a permanent or portable induction loop) which is well maintained, regularly tested, and for which appropriate staff training has been (and continues to be) given
- have a non-reflective glass screen (if one is provided)
- have additional, controllable, lighting which could be used to temporarily increase the light available for people with poor vision or reduced hearing
- have suitable general lighting for people who rely on lip reading
- be placed in an acoustic environment which exhibits low noise and reverberation
- have information in alternative formats (large print, audio tape etc).

10.4 Reception desks

10.4.1 Dimensions

The figure below shows the dimensions that will allow a wheelchair user to access and use a counter or reception desk. Wherever possible, there should be sufficient space and a moveable chair for a wheelchair user's companion to sit beside them. Where there are forms to be completed or documents to be signed, the counter or reception desk profile should have a knee and footrest recess to allow the wheelchair user to get as close to the counter or desk as possible. Control barriers must not reduce the manoeuvring space adjacent to the counter or desk.

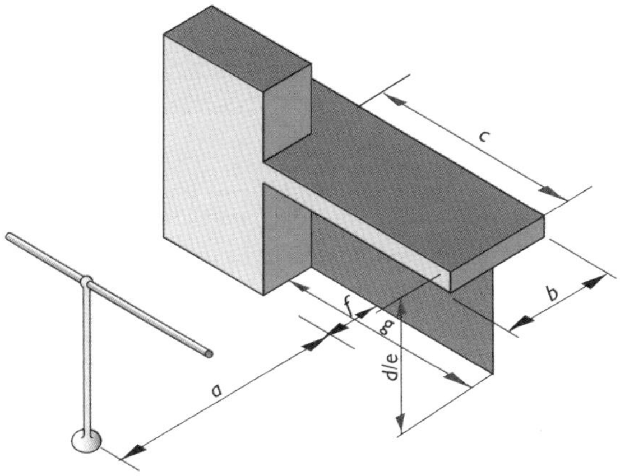

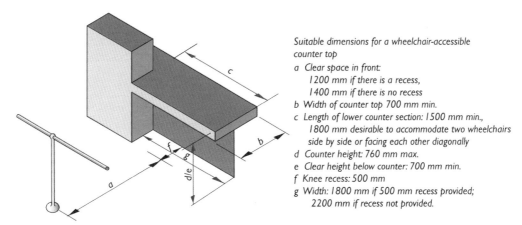

Suitable dimensions for a wheelchair-accessible counter top

a Clear space in front:
1200 mm if there is a recess,
1400 mm if there is no recess

b Width of counter top 700 mm min.

c Length of lower counter section: 1500 mm min., 1800 mm desirable to accommodate two wheelchairs side by side or facing each other diagonally

d Counter height: 760 mm max.

e Clear height below counter: 700 mm min.

f Knee recess: 500 mm

g Width: 1800 mm if 500 mm recess provided; 2200 mm if recess not provided.

Figure 10a Reception counter dimensions

10.4.2 Security

In some environments, there is serious potential conflict between making a counter or reception desk accessible, and maintaining an appropriate level of security or protection for staff working behind the desk. While this may be an obvious conflict for businesses such as financial institutions and government offices, it is becoming an increasing concern in other areas such as doctors' surgeries, employment offices and chemists. In such environments, lowering a counter or reception desk to improve accessibility will have to be considered against the need to provide security screens that will undoubtedly increase the cost of the improvement.

See 8.1.5

10.4.3 Induction loops

An induction loop should be fitted to all reception desks and counters where important information is to be discussed, for example at a pharmaceutical counter in a chemist's or hospital. However, the provision of an induction loop alone does not ensure that an employer, or service provider, has met the needs of all people who are deaf or hard of hearing, only those who use a hearing aid with a "T switch". (see also Chapter 5).

Installing an induction loop is not enough. It must also be fully operational at the time it is needed and staff must be fully trained to use it.

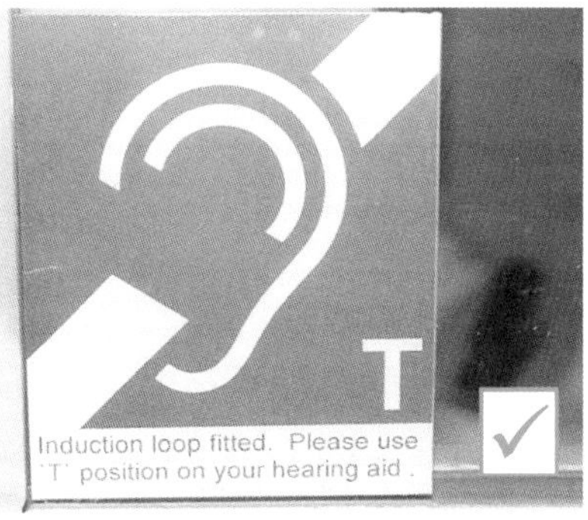

4. The sign that indicates an induction loop has been fitted. It is necessary to ensure that it is working when needed and that staff are appropriately trained in its use. Linking its provision to an ongoing maintenance programme, and moving quickly to repair it if necessary, is essential.

10.4.4 Staff training

Fully trained staff at counters and reception desks can considerably improve the perceived, and actual, accessibility of the whole building, and assist in addressing important security and safety issues. Staff should:

- be trained to meet the needs of disabled people and how to interact with them
- know of potential dangers or hazards which may affect them and be aware of what to do if necessary
- know where facilities such as accessible toilets are located, and know the easiest route to them
- undergo basic mobility training to assist people with visual impairments if required
- undergo basic training in clear lip speaking with some staff having a basic competence in sign language.

10.5 Issues about existing counters or reception desks

In an existing situation, understanding how the counter of a desk is actually used, can assist in the decision whether an immediate replacement of the counter or desk is needed, or whether features such as lowered sections can wait until the desk is next refurbished or replaced.

If form filling, signing, or writing are necessary at the counter of an existing desk, options that could be considered are:

- providing a small drop down shelf attached the front of the desk to give a suitable surface when needed
- providing another facility, such as an additional desk within the reception area, to be used by both disabled and non-disabled visitors and customers
- changing management practices to remove the need for signing in or writing.

A rail at the front of the counter or desk to assist those users who use walking aids or who experience difficulties with balance when standing still, should also be considered.

10.6 Waiting areas

10.6.1 Generally

Waiting areas should be comfortable, easy to use and designed to include and address the needs of disabled people. This can be done by:

- considering disabled people's needs when deciding on a queuing system, especially if within a bank of counters only one is adapted to meet their needs
- providing circulation routes where wheelchair users and other disabled people can wait with their companions
- providing a selection of good seating design that colour contrasts with the surroundings
- providing a combination of fixed and moveable seating which can accommodate a number of seating arrangements and numbers of people
- ensuring that waiting areas are in the view of the reception staff
- adopting management procedures which ensure that the time a person is required to stand is minimised and that sufficient time for standing up is given if necessary
- providing warm and well lit waiting areas (see Chapter 13).

See 14.7

10.6.2 Queuing

Disabled people can be at a disadvantage if a managed queuing system is not adopted. If a call system is being used, both visual and audible signals should be given. Queuing lanes should be wide enough to allow for wheelchairs, assistance dog users and people using crutches to wait and progress comfortably in the queue and to turn towards the counter or desk. There should be sufficient space for other users to pass behind them when they are using a counter or desk, or for the disabled person to turn around and leave the queue. A place should also be provided which is of sufficient size for one wheelchair to pass another.

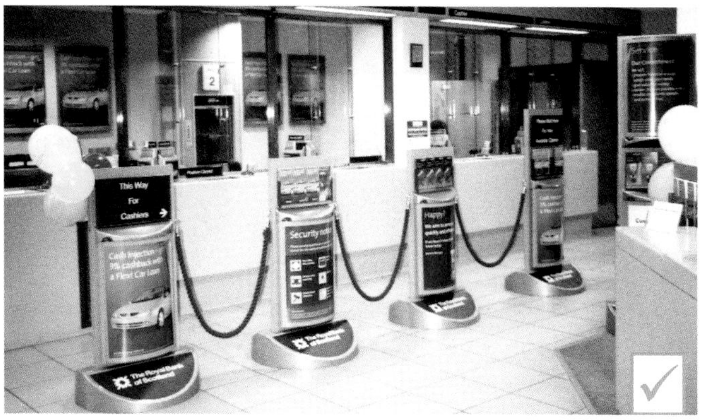

5. This is a good example of the use of ropes to highlight a queuing lane. They are not intended to be a permanent feature. However, the lane would not be wide enough for wheelchair users when they are trying to manoeuvre in front of the counter.

For people with visual impairments, a winding route defined by barriers can be very difficult to negotiate, especially if there is no low level tapping rail to assist mobility. If the route of the queue is along a wall or counter, it will be easier to follow. All barriers for demarcation of a queuing route should be robust and clearly differentiated from the surrounding area using colour and luminance contrast.

Rails should either be robust or clearly identifiable as not being intended to give support (eg ropes or tapes).

10.6.3 Seating

Access to seating in general waiting areas should be direct and unobstructed.

Seating should:

- be provided on a level surface
- have a variety of seat heights
- have a selection of seats with and without arms
- be robust enough, both in terms of the seat and the arms, to ensure that a disabled person is not at risk if they use the arms of the chair to assist them when sitting down or standing up
- incorporate some seats with high backs
- contrast in terms of colour and luminance with the surface against which it will be viewed. In smaller areas, this is likely to be the wall, but in larger areas it may be both the wall and the floor.
- have sufficient flexibility to allow two wheelchair or assistance dog users to sit next to each other, or for them to sit next to a companion who may or may not be disabled.

Spaces for use by wheelchair or assistance dog users should be designed into the layout, not simply provided on the edge of the area.

6. An example of a seating area where all the chairs are at the same height. The waste paper bin is causing an obstruction and the low headroom under the stairs is a dangerous problem for everybody.

   Good warning signage is required or, preferably, the seating area should be moved to a more suitable location.

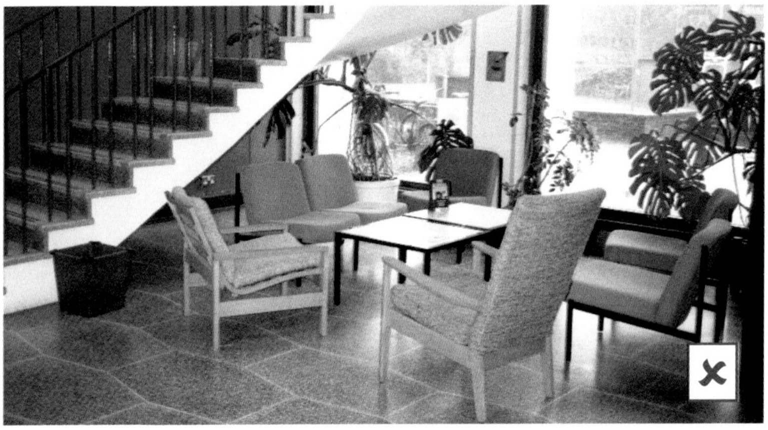

See 8.8.3, 16.9.1, 16.11.2, 16.11.3, 16.11.4

10.6.4 Ticket machines

Where queuing is organised by a ticket system, the ticket dispenser should be placed at a height that is accessible to both disabled and non-disabled users. Both visual and audible announcements of numbers being called must be given. Self service ticket machines and ATMs must also be suitable for independent use by disabled people.

See 8.5.3, 8.5.4

10.6.5 Restricted reception areas or arrivals spaces

Where the reception area or arrival space in an existing building is restricted and appropriate provision cannot be made for waiting, tickets can be issued and enquiries dealt with at another point, perhaps a kiosk, along the route. However, that provision, and its operation, must be fully accessible to disabled people.

In some restricted areas, it may be possible to provide fold down or perch seats to assist people who experience difficulty with standing or mobility.

If, in a restricted space, disabled people have to wait for the start of a tour or to be guided around a building, there should be space, perhaps in a separate area or building, where one or more persons can wait comfortably and without causing an obstruction.

10.7 Security

10.7.1 Turnstiles

Disabled people unable to use turnstiles must be provided with an accessible pass gate. Appropriate management practices and procedures must also be in place to ensure the ease of access into or out of the building is equal to that of other turnstile users.

See 10.2.1

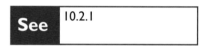

10.7.2 Other security doors

See Chapter 8 for details of other measures to be taken when considering security at the entrance or exit of a building.

11 Horizontal circulation

11.1 Design principles

11.1.1 Unimpeded movement

Horizontal circulation includes lobbies, corridors, horizontal movement within an assembly area or room, and any small change in level within the same floor. In buildings that are open totally or partially to the public, all users should be able to move around freely on a horizontal level without any barriers to physical access. This is also true in terms of reasonable adjustments to horizontal access to meet the specific access requirements of existing employees in their work environment. Any constraints placed upon a building in terms of facilitating evacuation, ensuring health and safety and required levels of security, should not compromise the ease of movement within and around a building.

11.1.2 Unobstructed routes

Lobbies and corridors should be kept free from obstacles and hazards such as radiators, fire extinguishers, hose reels, filing cabinets, furniture, public telephones, noise reduction screens and waste paper bins. Any existing obstacles should be recessed or placed so they do not impede the line of travel for people passing through a lobby or along a corridor. Staff training procedures should be introduced to ensure that that all horizontal routes are kept free from obstructions as a matter of course.

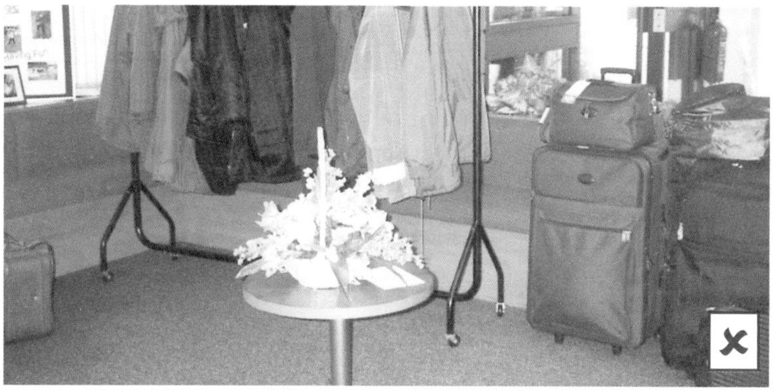

1. Wherever possible, areas off the circulation route should be allocated for the storage of everyday items. Here, there are too many potential hazards for many disabled people – and it doesn't look very attractive either.

11.1.3 Accessible information about a route

Horizontal routes can be confusing to a person who is unfamiliar with the building. Information to assist people navigate around a building can be given by:

- well designed and positioned signage
- tactile clues:
  - such as changes in floor surface coverings outside WCs, lifts etc
  - wall-mounted handrails with tactile directional dots
  - maps in both written and tactile formats
  - the use of different floor finishes to identify designated areas, for example in distinguishing circulation routes in large retail areas from sales areas
- lighting which directs people along a route
- colour and contrast to differentiate routes and areas
- aromas
- audible clues, for example a fountain or water feature.

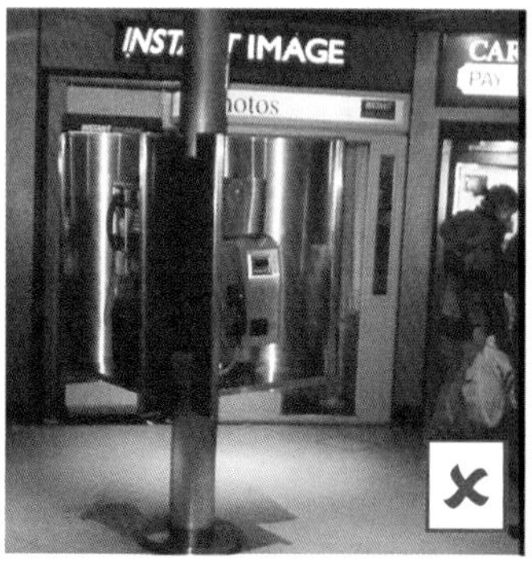

2. Facilities projecting into circulation routes, such as the telephones here, are a serious potential hazard for many users, but especially those with poor vision. The reflective surfaces mean they blend into their surroundings, and people with a visual impairment who use mobility aids, such as long canes, are unlikely to detect the presence of the projection before colliding with it.

For some users, air movement can also give valuable information about which direction to take.

11.2 Strategy for existing buildings

11.2.1 Use of space

Access within existing buildings can be restricted or limited by narrow corridors, constrained lobby areas, cramped toilet accommodation and changes in the actual floor level within the same floor. When refurbishing an existing building it is often possible to alter original features and reorganise or incorporate existing or wasted space to provide accessible toilet facilities, ramps, platform lifts, wider corridors and larger lobbies. By adopting good design practice, it is also feasible to remove intermediate changes in floor level which previously would have affected horizontal circulation within an existing building. However, it is essential that the structural stability of the building is not affected by any proposed modifications.

See 9.2.2, 9.3.4, 9.6.5, 10.2.1, 10.2.2, 10.6.5, 11.6.1, 12.6.5, 12.6.7

11.2.2 Improvement within normal maintenance

Some improvements to an existing building can be undertaken as part of the routine maintenance and management procedures. Such changes could include:

- improving signage
- upgrading or simply increasing/decreasing lighting
- replacing floor surfaces to incorporate wayfinding or tactile information detectable underfoot
- internal redecoration to reflect good use of colour and tonal contrast
- changing vision panels when upgrading internal fire doors
- partial or total rewiring to relocate or increase the number of controls available.

Routine maintenance and operation of the building can be programmed in order to make circulation routes safer... for example, cleaning light fittings regularly, washing floors when the building is not in use, and closing window blinds in bright sunshine to minimise glare.

11.2.3 Management procedures

Staff training is essential and should be provided on a regular basis. Key staff should be familiar with the operation and maintenance of equipment such as lifts, stairlifts and platform lifts, and emergency evacuation procedures including location of safe refuges and Evac chairs.

See 12.5.1, 12.6, 12.7, 12.8, 15.12.2.

11.3 Corridors and lobbies

11.3.1 Corridor requirements

Corridors should:

Visibility

- avoid reflective surfaces
- have minimal glare or shadow from natural light
- have good, relatively even, interior lighting.

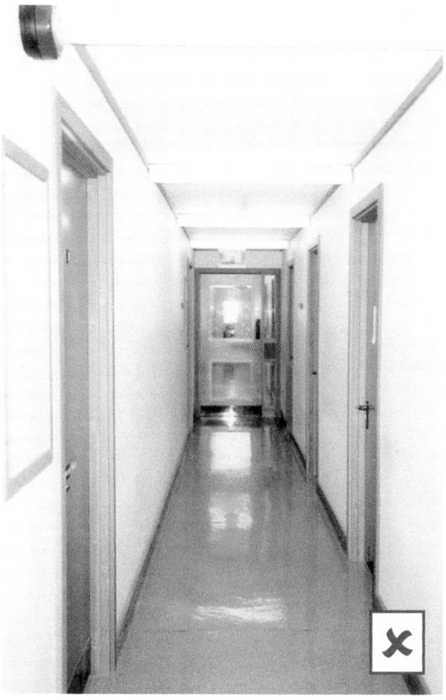

3 & 4. Reflective floor finishes are bad for people with visual impairments, older people and people who use mobility aids because they perceive them as wet and therefore, potentially slippery. Providing a non-reflective floor surface, in this case short pile carpet, provides a much more helpful environment, often at little or no additional cost. Shame about the poor vision panels, but a good use of handrails and tactile flooring to alert people of the presence of the doors.

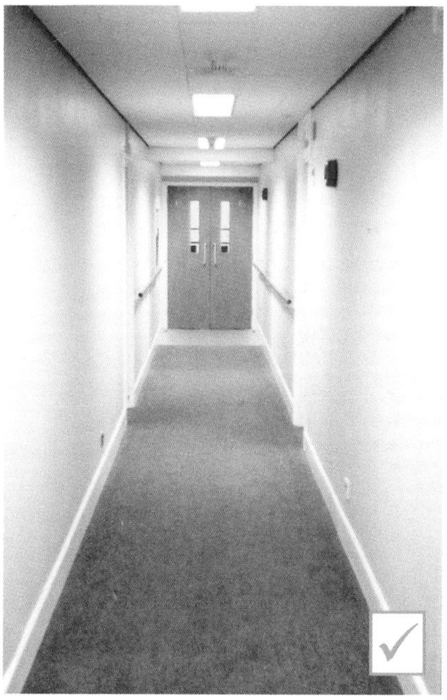

Ease of approach

- be fitted with handrails on both sides of a corridor when required, such as when there is a change in level that has a steep gradient
- have a level surface or be provided with a ramp/platform lift at changes in floor level.

Usability

- be wide enough for wheelchair users to manoeuvre and provide adequate space for passing side by side
- be colour-contrasted to highlight features, for example, light sockets, skirting boards, door handles and architraves or to identify different corridors or floor levels
- be provided with passing places in narrow corridors at reasonable intervals to assist wheelchair users in manoeuvring.

Good communication

- be provided with tactile clues on handrails (if appropriate) to warn of changes in level or the approach of a step
- have appropriately positioned, easy-to-read and well contrasted signage, particularly directional signage and exit signs (see Chapter 5).

Safety of use

- have a slip-resistant and firm floor surface
- not have busy, patterned or deep pile floor surface coverings
- have firmly fixed carpet with no loose edges
- be free from obstacles, obstructions and any projections
- have vision panels in doors along main corridor routes
- avoid fully-glazed doors across main corridor routes
- be provided with protective angles/strips at corners of walls and skirtings
- have kick plates to protect doors along corridors
- not have doors which open into the corridor/circulation route – with the exception of toilet doors and doors to service ducts.

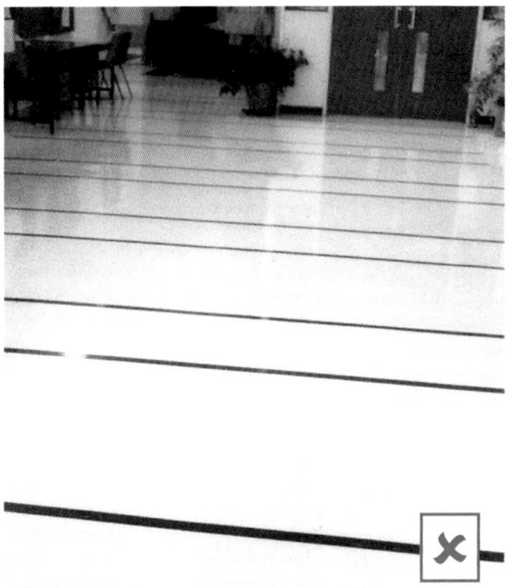

5. The floor pattern (left) may be viewed as a series of steps to people with impaired vision. They will be hesitant when navigating through this space.
6. The damage on this door could have been avoided by the use of kick plates.

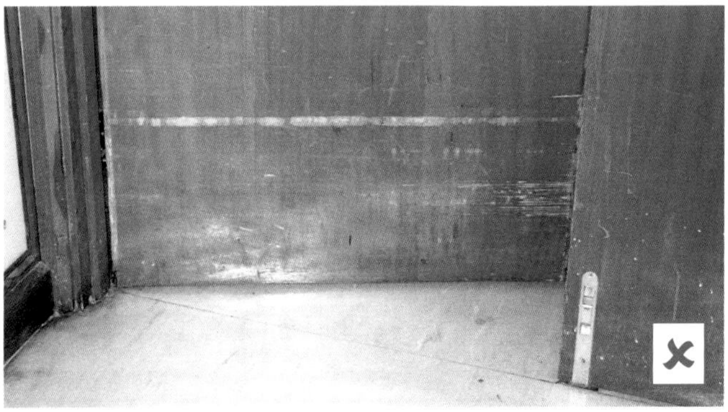

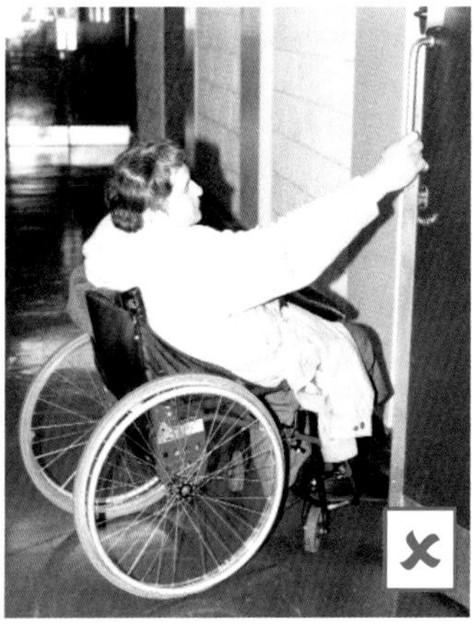

7. Simply lengthening the "D-shaped" door handle would make this door much more accessible for everyone, and it could be done at very little additional cost.

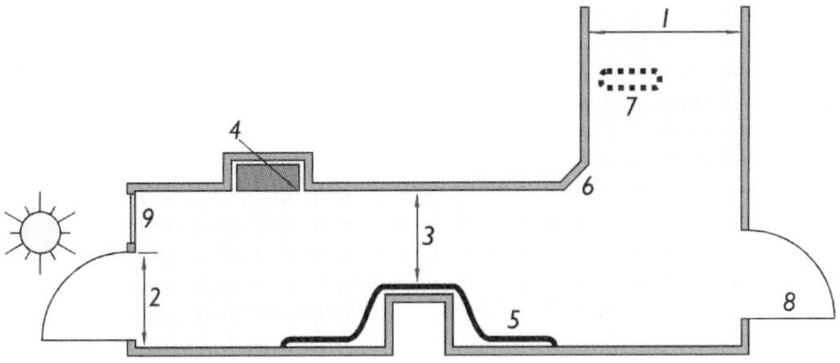

Key
1 1800 mm width for two wheelchairs to pass
2 750 mm min., 800 mm preferred, clear width for head-on wheelchair approach through a door
3 1200 mm min. clear width of corridor or 1000 mm min. clear width where there is a permanent restriction over a short distance. If corridor is likely to be used frequently by wheelchair users the clear width of the corridor should be 1800 mm or passing places of length 1800 mm min. should be provided at reasonable intervals.
4 Recess fittings (e.g. use blocked-up door opening o r recess)
5 Unavoidable projections should be guarded (e.g. with handrail)
6 Splay or round corners to give more space
7 Avoid overhead signs that people could collide with
8 Doors in corridors should open into room. Avoid outward-opening doors
9 Avoid glass panels that people could collide with –and avoid brightly lit glazing at end of corridor – glare can make seeing much more difficult for some partially sighted people.

Figure 11a Dimensions and design of corridors

11.3.2 Narrow corridors

Circulation routes in existing buildings may be narrower than the dimensions recommended in BS 8300 and other design guidance. If this is the case, it is necessary to plan corridor spaces so that wheelchairs can manoeuvre as easily as possible. This may be achieved by introducing passing places if possible or utilising space in adjacent rooms that would allow some space for wheelchairs to pass. However, such arrangements must only be used in cases of occasional access where it is not possible to provide full width corridors. In no circumstances should a corridor that is to be used for wheelchair access be less than 800 mm wide. In any corridor less than 1800 mm wide, passing places should be provided.

11.3.3 Internal lobby requirements

Internal lobbies should be designed and be managed to have:

- appropriate space and positioning of doors to allow satisfactory manoeuvring by a wheelchair user
- door closers adjusted to minimum force necessary and regularly maintained
- firmly fixed floor coverings and no loose door mats or sunken mat wells.

See 9.6.2, 11.1.1, 11.1.2, 11.3.1

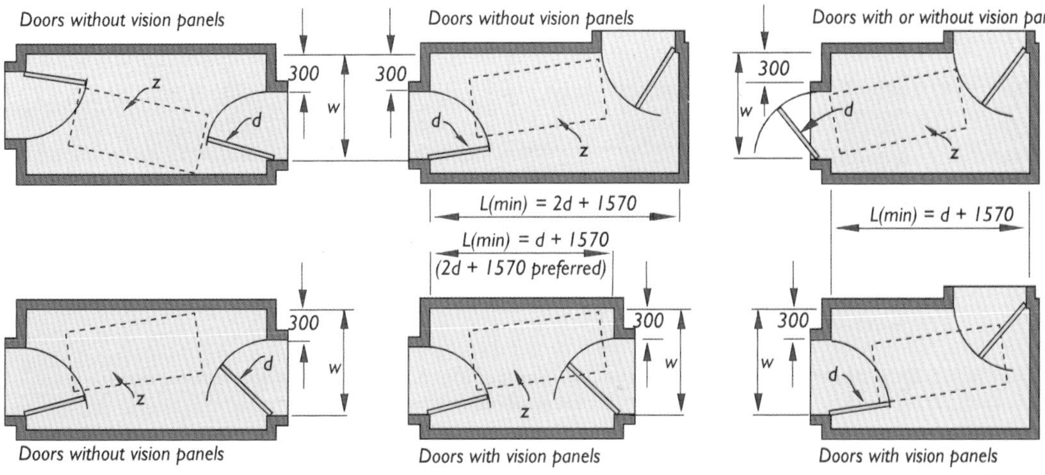

Key
L = Length of lobby
d = Width of door leaf
z = 1570 mm by 750 mm zone for wheelchair accompanied by an attendant
w = (d = 300) or 1200 mm, whichever is greater

Dimensions in mm

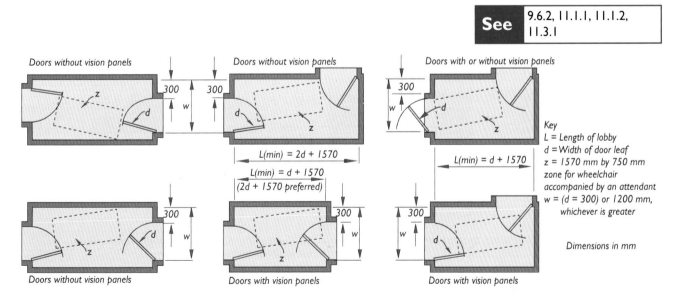

Figure 11b Minimum dimensions of lobbies with single leaf doors.

11.4 Doors – internal

11.4.1 General design principles

General design principles for doors are given in Chapter 9.6. The additional issues specifically related to internal doors are given here.

Internal doors should:

- have a minimum clear opening width of 750 mm (with a preference for 800 mm wherever possible). Where there are two leaves to a door, at least one of the leaves should have a clear opening width of 750 mm (800 mm preferred).
- not be fully-glazed, especially if they are situated across main corridor routes.

In some existing buildings, it may be necessary to replace doors that are of equal width (but each less than 750 mm) with doors of unequal width (a "door and half set"). The leaf that has a clear opening width of at least 750 mm (800 mm preferred), must be the leaf that is most likely to be used by people passing along the corridor.

Automatically operated and power assisted doors are easier to use for everyone, including wheelchair users and people with mobility impairments. Automatic sliding doors can be used to increase the amount of lobby space available in an existing building. Automatic door operators can be fitted to most doors in existing buildings.

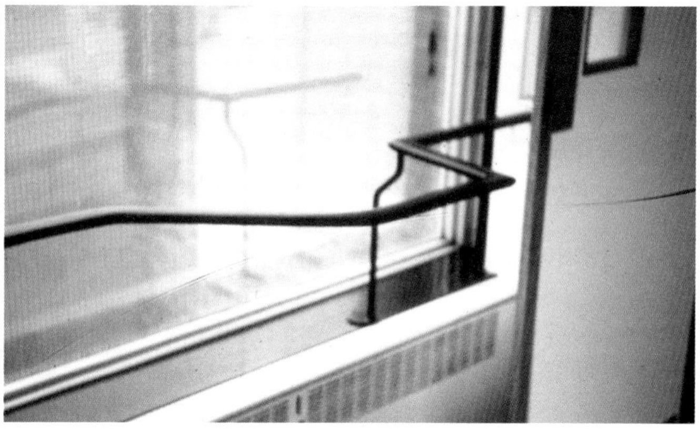

8. If doors must project into the circulation route, then open, handrails can be used to advise users of the potential danger. The leading edge of the door should be highlighted with colour and luminance contrast.

See 9.6.1, 9.6.9

11.4.2 Dimensions

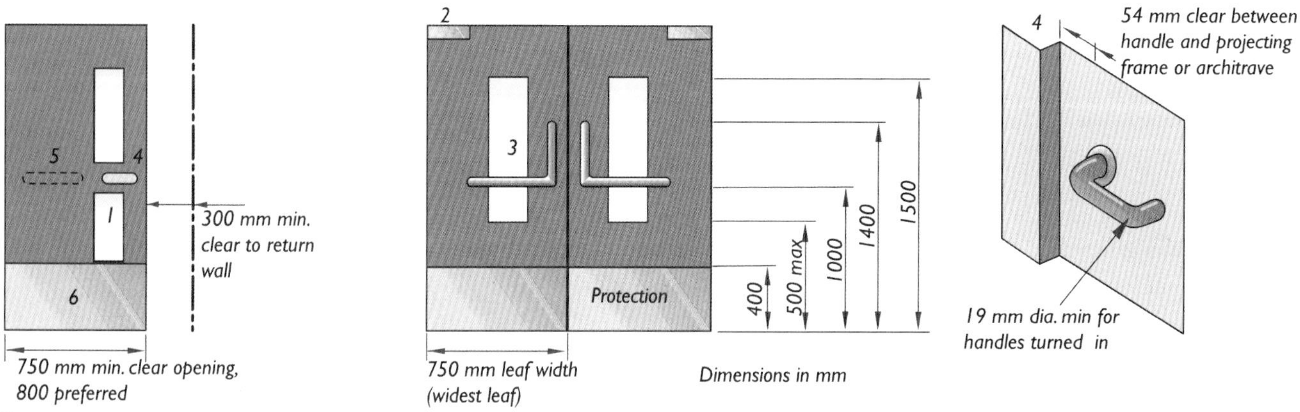

Key

1 Vision panel for wheelchair users (where privacy is not required)
2 Closers that can be adjusted to require minimum opening force and to close slowly
3 Vertical and horizontal push-and-pull handles
4 Easily gripped lever handles suited to push-and-pull operation
5 Extra pull handle where space allows
6 Protection against marks and denting from wheelchair footrests

Figure 11c Design of manually operated doors

A door-closing device for security, privacy or energy control should not exceed 20N.

11.4.3 Manually operated doors

Manually operated doors should be designed for use by everyone, but with particular consideration to wheelchair users, people with vision impairments and people with limited manual dexterity.

11.4.4 Ironmongery

Hinges

Single axis hinges should conform to the requirements of BS 7352 (BS 8300: 2001 page 33). The position of fixed hinges should conform to the requirements of BS 4787:1. Hinges with low fraction bearings should be used when it is necessary to minimise door opening and closing forces. Cranked or projecting hinges can sometimes be used to increase the existing door width.

Handles

When choosing door furniture, it is essential to ensure that it has smooth operation, provides a secure grip and is correctly positioned for easy reach.

The minimum recommended diameter of handles is 19 mm. This measurement is of critical importance to disabled people, and especially those people with manual dexterity impairments.

Wherever possible, door-opening furniture with a lever handle should be used. Door furniture with spherical, circular or similar designed doorknobs, can be difficult for many people to use, but especially for disabled people and older people with restricted manual strength or dexterity. It should be possible to operate the door-opening furniture with one hand, without grasping it or twisting the wrist. All door furniture should contrast in colour and/or luminance with the surface of the door, for easy identification by people with a visual impairment.

Wherever possible, door furniture should exceed the recommended minimum lever diameter of 19 mm. This will help to ensure that there is sufficient material in the handle to make operation easier. Narrow styles can be painful to grip for people with arthritis.

Round bar furniture is preferred because it does not have sharp edges. It should also have a return to the door to help prevent hands slipping off the end of the lever, or loose clothing being caught. For secure use, bolt-through fixing is essential.

As some disabled people may lean heavily on door furniture for physical support, the lever itself must be suitable, both in design and materials, to be robust in use.

See 16.3.3

Locks and latches

Where a lock is required in conjunction with a lever handle, an upright mortice lock/latch should be used.

To ensure that people with a visual impairment or restricted dexterity have unobstructed access to the keyway, the cylinder should either be above the lever handle, or have a minimum distance of 72 mm between the handle and the keyway of the locking mechanism. It is important that the latchbolt should have an easy action, ensuring that closing forces can be kept to a minimum, which will result in lower opening forces.

11.5 Changes of level within a storey

11.5.1 Bypassing steps

If steps impede the horizontal movement within an existing building for any user, an alternative option should be provided such as a platform lift or the addition of a ramp. Only when an alternative provision is not possible, should the steps be completely replaced with a ramp.

11.5.2 Single steps

Single steps are often found in existing buildings, particularly where a property may have been extended or modified. If this cannot be avoided, the step should be highlighted with a contrasting nosing and well lit. A portable ramp or set of articulated tracks may be a solution for wheelchair users in overcoming a single step within a storey, provided there is a management procedure in place to provide assistance with any kind of portable ramp.

See 9.3.1

11.6 Ramps

11.6.1 Space for ramps

The main problem with incorporating a ramp to overcome a change in level in an existing corridor is lack of suitable space. The most obvious solutions are to utilise space from adjoining rooms, cupboards and light wells. There may be consequences for the building in carrying out this type of work, such as a reduction in room space, lower lighting levels or loss of storage space.

11.6.2 Doors adjacent to ramps

If the only location for a ramp coincides with an existing door opening, there are two options available: firstly, blocking up the existing door and creating an alternative door opening in a more suitable location or, secondly, raising the level of the floor within the room to which the door provides access so that it is on the same level as the intermediate landing of the ramp.

11.6.3 Ramp replacing a single step

If a single step is replaced by a ramp, the location of the ramp should be clearly identified by the use of colour or tonal contrast for all users, but particularly those with ambulant or balance problems. It is good practice to provide handrails.

11.7 Floor surfaces

11.7.1 Floor surface requirements

Floor surfaces should:

Visibility

- not have high gloss finishes.

Ease of approach

- be firmly fixed, particularly at entrances and changes in level
- be easy to navigate and avoid the use of high resistant floor coverings, such as deep pile carpets and coir matting.

Usability

- not be covered with large and repeating patterns, which may be perceived as steps by people with visual impairments.

Good communication

- incorporate the use of colour contrast to highlight junctions of floors with walls, doors, columns and barriers (BS 4800 in conjunction with BS 5252)
- maximise the use of textured surfaces to provide clues for navigation (Ref: Department for Transport, Mobility and Inclusion Unit: *Guidance on the use of tactile paving surfaces*)
- conform to the recommendations for acoustic design given in BS 8233.

Safety of use

- be level and slip resistant
- not be covered with loose door mats and rugs.

See 5.4

11.7.2 Appearance

Indiscriminate changes of floor finish, patterns, colour and luminance contrast, and reflectivity, can be confusing for all users, but especially for older people and people with visual impairments. Sharp changes in colour can falsely indicate the presence of a step.

Shiny surfaces can appear to be wet and hence slippery, both of which are potentially dangerous conditions for people with mobility impairments, or who use aids such as crutches and sticks. They may be uncertain, feel very uncomfortable when walking on them, and may well refuse to make the journey at all. Floor finishes that are highly reflective should be avoided.

12 Vertical circulation

It is when wishing to travel vertically within an environment that many disabled people will experience the most difficult problems with access. It is probably also the most difficult problem owners and managers of existing buildings will face in trying to improve the overall accessibility of their building or environment. There are many potential solutions to improving manual or assisted vertical travel but what is important is to choose the method most appropriate to users while bearing in mind constraints imposed by the existing structure of the building.

12.1 Design principles

12.1.1 All floors accessible

All floors of an existing building should be available and accessible to all users. The only exceptions are sections of the building where access is required only for the maintenance of plant and machinery.

To reduce the risk of tripping or losing balance, all internal changes in level, including single steps and short ramps, should be clearly identified.

12.1.2 Independent access

All users of an existing building should be able to access all floors of that building independently. It should not be necessary for disabled people to be accompanied when using lifts, stair lifts, platform lifts, stairs or escalators.

Ramps and/or lifts should be provided at all changes of level for people who are unable to use, or prefer not to use, stairs.

See 5.2.2, 9.1.1, 9.2.2

12.1.3 Safe, easy to use and operate

All items of equipment used to assist vertical circulation within an existing building should be safe and easy to use and operate. The location of stairs, lifts and escalators should be clearly identified by the use of appropriate signage. Clear and concise instructions should be available in an alternative format where appropriate, and management procedures should ensure that relevant staff have been trained to assist all users if the equipment fails for any reason. Lifts, platform lifts, stairlifts and escalators should be regularly maintained by the appropriate manufacturer.

12.2 Strategy for existing buildings

12.2.1 Advantages of passenger lifts

The provision of an accessible user-friendly lift can have a major impact on the accessibility of an existing building or an environment. For many disabled people passenger lifts are the preferred means of vertical circulation within an existing building. However, the installation of this type of lift places the most demand on the existing structure in terms of space required for a lift shaft and the disturbance and noise resulting from the installation work.

The only time a passenger lift may not be suitable is when an existing building has been constructed using mezzanine floors on half levels between floors and it is not possible to install a lift to serve intermediate floor levels. In such cases, the only alternative may be to install a platform stairlift which can serve these intermediate floors.

When deciding upon the location of a lift in an existing building, consideration must be given to how the existing space is used. If space is at a premium and the amount of existing space is essential for the operation of that building, it may be possible to utilise existing stair voids, or construct an external lift shaft to incorporate the new lift.

See 6.3.3, 12.5, 12.5.1, 15.6.3

12.2.2 Lift costs

The cost of installing a passenger lift is greater than that for a platform stairlift, but the advantages and disadvantages of each piece of equipment should be weighed up against each other by the operator of the existing building. If the building has a limited life, or is occupied on a short-term tenancy basis, a platform stairlift may be the best solution, particularly if the existing building has only a few upper floors. However, if the building is occupied on a long lease and has a large number of upper floors, a passenger lift may be the preferred option. Even though this may be a costly improvement, the benefits of improving accessibility for all users may well outweigh the cost involved.

12.2.3 Implications of accessibility

If the upper floors of an existing building are made accessible to all users of that building, it is essential to consider evacuation procedures in the case of an emergency, when the lift cannot be used. There will be a need for a refuge area, appropriate signage and staff training procedures. (see Chapter 15). Other facilities will also have to be considered, such as the incorporation of additional accessible toilet facilities on upper floors.

12.2.4 Existing lifts and stairs

In existing buildings, even if a lift is already installed, it may not meet the spatial requirements and other recommendations in BS 8300: 2001. However, it may be possible to adjust some items quite easily, such as the existing heights of controls and handrails, and fitting tactile embossed and Braille legends over existing lift control panels to assist people with visual impairments. If the lift car is too small for wheelchair users, the only alternative may be to install a new lift at a time of refurbishment, although a careful examination of the management practices affecting how the building is used, may well negate the need for access to upper floors in some situations. Installing a new lift, if required, is likely to be the most expensive item of any refurbishment work.

Existing staircases may also not conform to the recommendations of BS 8300: 2001. While it may be possible to resurface treads, incorporate nosings and alter or provide new handrails with the minimum of disruption and cost, changing the existing stair profile in terms of tread and rise dimensions will not be a practical proposition and this work will have to be done at the date of the next refurbishment. If an existing staircase has open risers, it may be possible to fit an upstand at the rear of each tread to improve safety and avoid the risk of tripping.

12.3 Steps and stairs

Steps and stairs are the most common way of providing access between changes in level and must be designed for safe and easy use by everyone. For disabled people, issues concerning stairs revolve around the suitability of handrails for tactile and physical support, good stair design and visibility.

Designs which incorporate projecting nosings, which can trap toes or callipers, and open risers, which can be very visually confusing for people with a visual impairment, should be avoided.

Handrails should be provided regardless of the number of steps.

The design of stairs should never present a danger to anyone using a building. Where there is access under the stairs or a projecting section, such as a half landing, the underside should be protected to prevent users, especially people with a visual impairment, from colliding with it.

1. A projecting half-landing with no protection to the underside. The underside of the landing is about 1.5 m affl and is on a route to the lifts.

A modern building with an in-built accident waiting to happen.

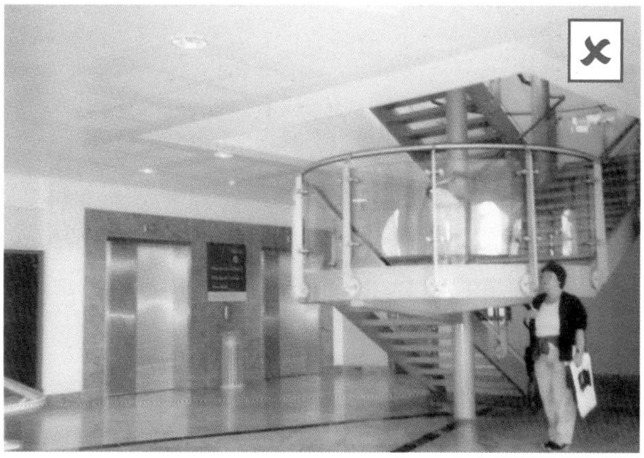

See 6.3.3, 9.2.1, 9.2.2, 9.3, 9.4, 11.5, 15.2

12.3.1 Internal step and stair requirements

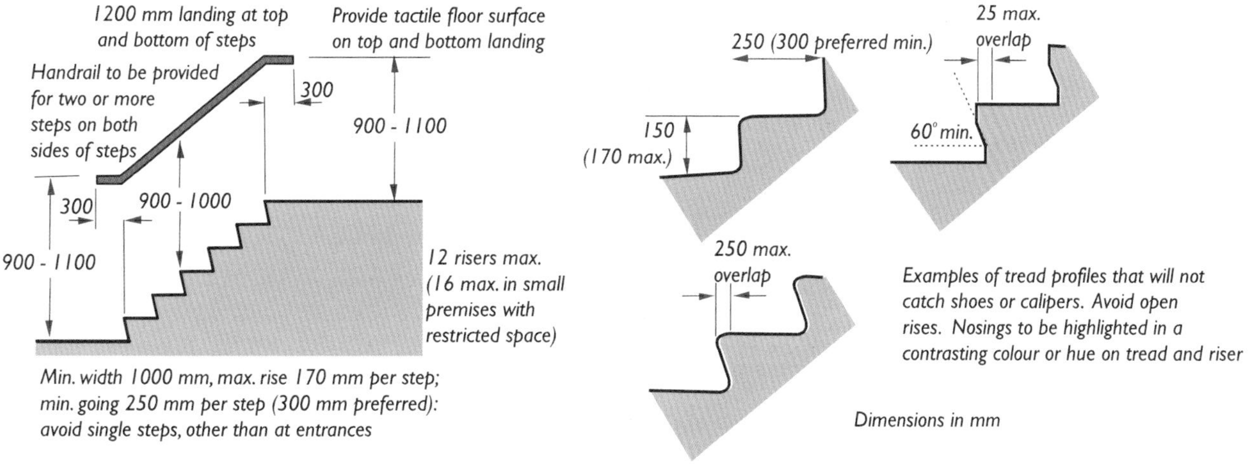

Figure 12a Internal stairs

Generally, steps and stairs should:

Visibility

- incorporate lighting at tread level of at least 100 lux
- have well-illuminated flights and landings
- avoid lighting which causes glare.

Ease of approach

- have a going width (tread width) of between 250 mm and 300 mm, but preferably 300 mm
- have a riser height between 150 mm and 170 mm maximum
- have dimensions so that the sum of the going (g) plus twice the rise (r) (ie g+2r) is between 550 mm and 700 mm
- have uniform goings within a staircase
- have a clear step width of 1000 mm minimum

- have a uniform number of risers in successive flights
- avoid the use of single isolated steps
- contain no more than 12 risers in a flight (except for smaller premises with restricted plan areas, where a maximum of 16 risers is allowed)
- conform to BS 5395-1: 2000 for the design of straight and winding stairs
- incorporate a level landing at least 1200 mm in length at the top and bottom of each flight of steps or stairs.

Usability

- have a uniform rise for each step within a flight and within a series of flights
- have slip-resistant treads (refer to BS 5395-1: 2000 guidance on slip-resistant surfaces).

Good communication

- have nosings which contrast in colour and luminance. Contrast should wrap around the nosing 40 mm on the riser and 40 mm on the going.
- incorporate a tactile warning positioned at least 400 mm from the nosing on the top landing of a flight of stairs.

Safety of use

- always be provided with a guard on the underside to prevent anyone colliding with the stair
- avoid open risers
- avoid tapered treads or spiral designs (especially in public access buildings)
- avoid projecting nosings (if nosings do project over the tread, this dimension should not exceed 25mm)
- incorporate balustrades which conform to BS 6180: 1999
- incorporate easy to maintain and slip-resistant floor surfaces.

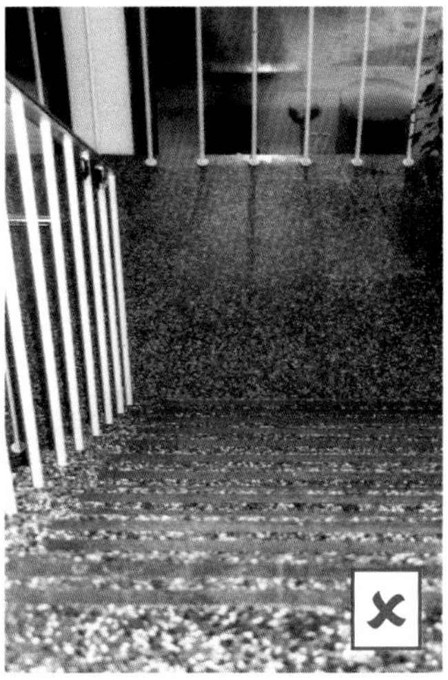

2. Poorly contrasted nosings, as seen here, can have a major impact on the ability of people to use the stairs safely. This is particularly so for people with a visual impairment.

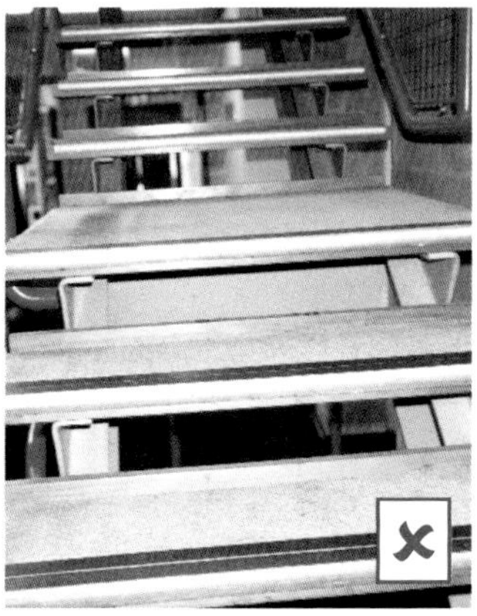

3. Open tread risers can cause confusion for people with visual impairments when ascending the stairs. People who use mobility aids such as long canes often experience difficulties with open risers as do people with restricted mobility and people who wear leg callipers.
The provision of open riser stairs should be avoided.

12.4 Handrails

Handrails are used for a variety of reasons when ascending or descending a stair, and the design and positioning of handrails is critical for many disabled people. People with a visual impairment use handrails for tactile clues, including when the steps start and finish, and for changes in direction. Some disabled people will use the handrails for physical support, and all users will need to use them if they trip or fall when using the stairs. Robust fittings are essential.

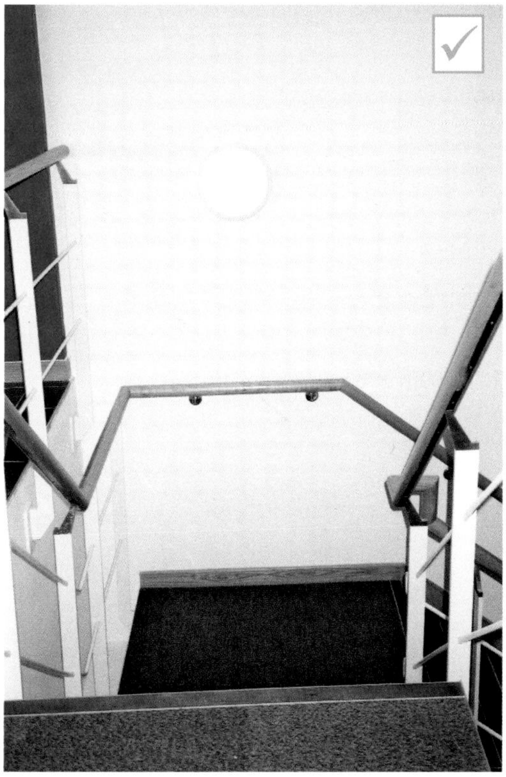

4. Continuous handrails around landings and good profile, both of which are good practice. Good colour and luminance contrast.

Handrails should be provided on both sides of a flight of steps, wherever possible. Wider flights of stairs can be divided with a central handrail, or a series of handrails.

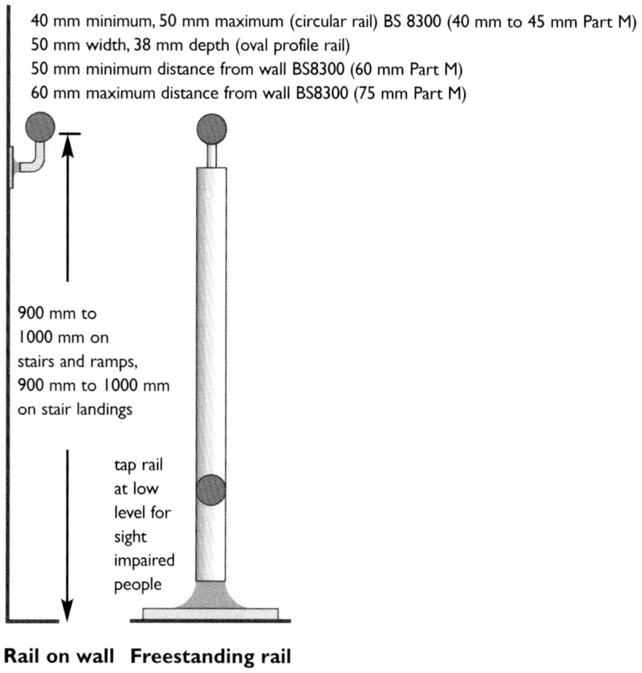

Figure 12b Handrail dimensions

The recommended dimensions for handrails are 40 mm – 50 mm if circular in design and 50 mm × 38 mm if oval. Handrails should extend 300 mm horizontally beyond the top and bottom of the steps and have positive ends. The horizontal extension allows for a person to gain information about the presence of a stair when it begins to ascend or descend, and to gain support before using the stairs. The positive end assists in reducing the risk of clothing being caught as the handrail is approached.

Handrails should contrast in terms of colour and luminance with the surrounding area, and be continuous around all landings and half landings.

It is good practice to provide surface coatings on handrails that are warm to the touch.

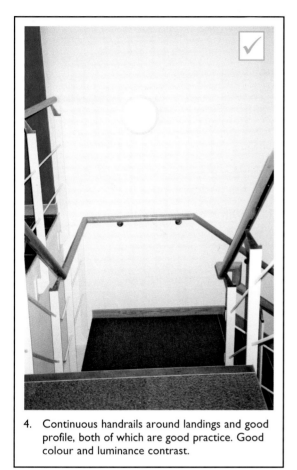

12.4.1 Handrail requirements

Handrails should:

Visibility

- be clearly visible, for example by the use of colour or tactile clues.

Ease of approach

- be positioned at a height of between 900 mm and 1000 mm above the pitch line of a flight of steps, when measured vertically
- be positioned at a height of between 900 mm and 1100 mm above the landing, when mentioned vertically
- incorporate an additional handrail where the clear width of the stairs exceeds 1800 mm and the stairs are used simultaneously by large numbers of people (the channel width created by the additional handrail should be between 1000 mm and 1800 mm)
- be positioned at a clear distance from the wall of between 50 mm and 60 mm
- extend horizontally at least 300 mm beyond the first and last nosing and return to the wall or have a positive end.

Usability

- be easy to grip
- have an appropriate cross sectional shape.

Good communication

- have tactile markers at the beginning and end of a flight indicating the floor level reached.

Safety of use

- be provided continuously on both sides of a flight of steps or stairs which comprise two or more risers
- be provided continuously around landings or half landings where staircases comprise two or more flights.

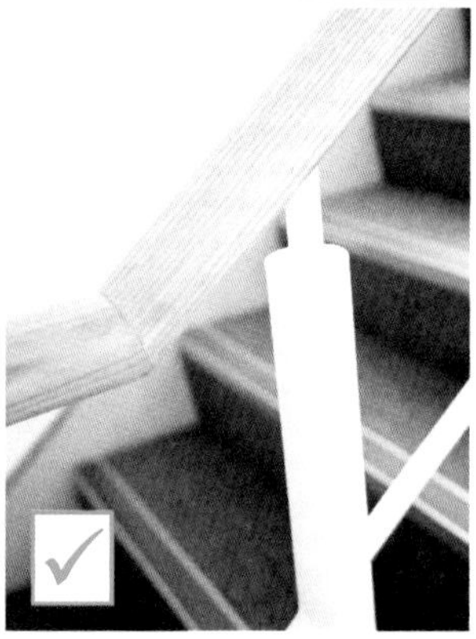

5. Good detailing of the handrail support to the handrail. The upright support should never be the same diameter as the handrail as this can cause injury to some disabled people when gripping and when sliding their hand along the handrail.

12.4.2 Existing handrails

In existing buildings, a practical compromise may have to be reached between the recommendations of BS 8300: 2001 and what is feasible on an existing staircase within the building. Safety of users must always be of paramount importance.

12.5 Passenger lifts

The location, number, and size of lifts in an existing building should be suitable to meet expected demand and type of building. In public access buildings, two lifts would allow for accessibility to be maintained if one is out of action for repair or maintenance. If only one lift is provided, management procedures must consider what action will be taken if it is temporarily out of commission.

The position of lifts should be clearly identified and there should be sufficient manoeuvring space outside the lift, which must be kept clear at all times. Existing lift cars that are smaller than the recommended minimum (1100 mm × 1400 mm), may still be suitable for a wheelchair user if the lift controls are accessible, or if assistance is given. In the longer term, however, lifts of a suitable size should be provided wherever possible.

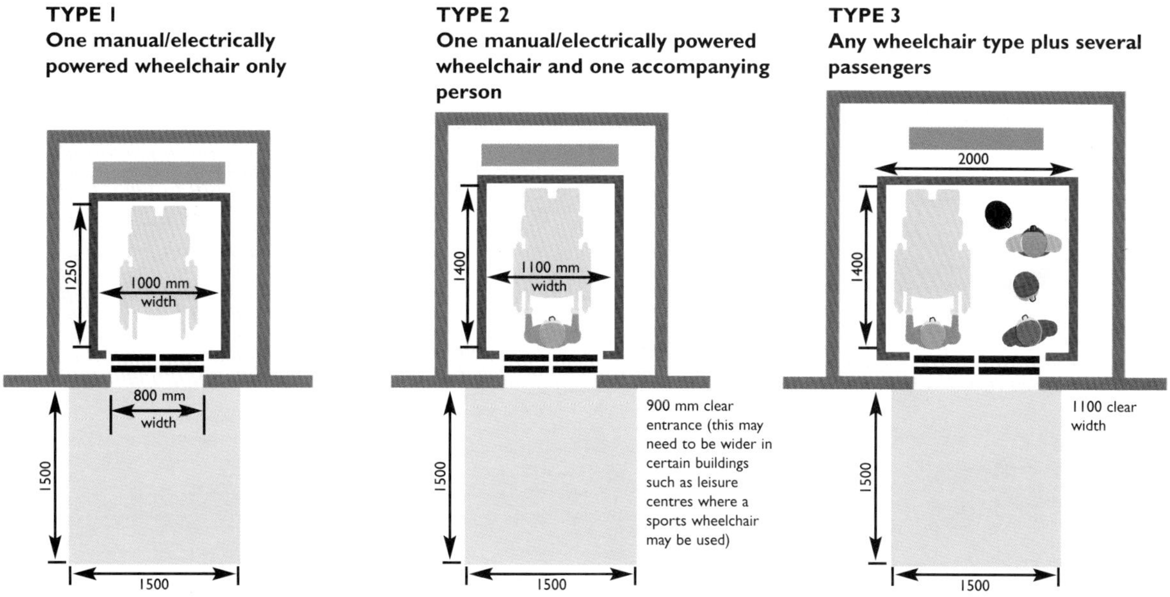

Electric lift installations from BSEN81-70:2003 showing minimum dimensions of lift car and landing for wheelchair use.

Figure 12c Standard lift sizes and dimensions

12.5.1 Passenger lifts

Passenger lifts should serve all floors in a multi-storey building and be of sufficient size to be accessible by wheelchair users and people with mobility problems (see Figure 12c). Lifts should conform to the requirements of BSEN81-70:2003 *Safety rules for the construction and installations of lifts*, which has particular applications for passenger and goods passenger lifts on "accessibility to lifts for persons including persons with disability".

Passenger lifts should also have:

Visibility

- clearly visible signage to identify the location of the lift
- a lift landing area with an illuminance of 100 lux minimum
- uniformly distributed lighting within the lift car at a level of 100 lux minimum, measured at floor level
- no vertical or horizontal lighting adjacent to control panels, which can cause glare
- non-reflective matt finishes to the lift car which contrast in colour and tone with the lift floor.

Ease of approach and exit

- a clear manoeuvring space of 1500 mm × 1500 mm in front of the lift car entrance, in a distinguishable floor surface
- a minimum clear entrance width to the lift car of 900 mm
- lift doors that when opened leave enough time to enter and exit the lift safely without the door closing onto passengers
- a mirror opposite the entrance of the lift car to assist wheelchair users when manoeuvring in and out of the lift. The mirror should not extend down below 900 mm affl
- a firm and slip-resistant lift floor surface.

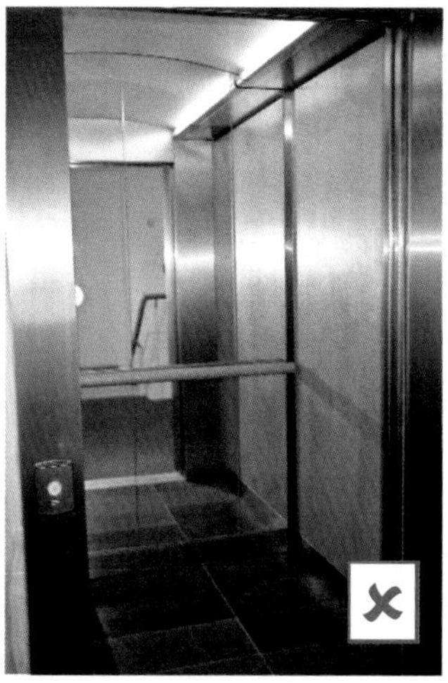

6. The mirror in this lift will cause confusion for people with a visual impairment because it is full height. Mirrors should not extend down below the handrail.

Usability

- lift control buttons located between 900 mm and 1100 mm (affl)
- lift control buttons fixed at a minimum distance of 400 mm from a return wall
- markings for each lift above the landing of each lift door.

Good communication

- visible and audible information for users when entering the lift car
- visible and audible signal confirmation for chosen floor selection
- audible information for users when the lift stops at each floor
- lift call buttons that contrast in colour and tone when viewed against their background
- tactile lift call buttons with embossed letters and numbers and Braille
- signs indicating the number of the floor on each lift landing on the wall opposite the lift
- a bell, intercom or external telephone which can be used in an emergency and a visual indicator to confirm that an emergency call has been recognised.

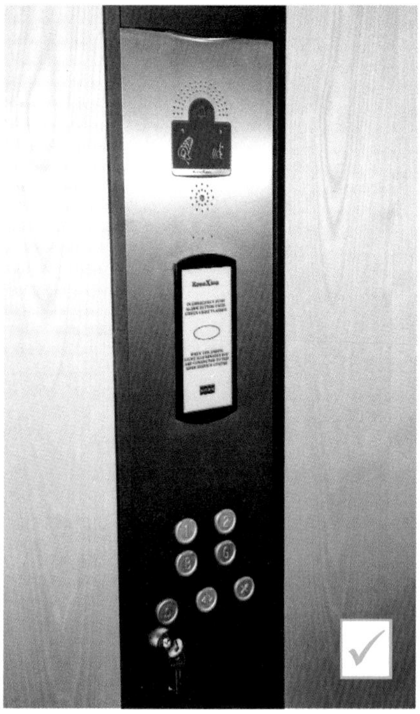

7. Good panel with tactile controls, photoluminescent signs (although the text is small) and a microphone that will detect sound without a handset. The red light that illuminates to indicate that the call has been received is also good practice.

Safety of use

- a minimum dwell time of five seconds after the doors have opened
- a handrail
- an independent power supply for evacuation in an emergency
- a provision for escape stairs for use in an emergency.

12.5.2 Standard design features

Table 12a Lift sizes and accommodation for users

Minimum car dimensions	Users who can be accommodated
Type 1 - BSEN81-70: 2003 1000 mm width and 1250 mm depth opening door width min 800 mm	One wheelchair user (manual or electrically powered chair) with no companion.
Type 2 - BSEN81-70: 2003 1100 mm width by 1400 mm depth opening door width min 900 mm	One wheelchair user (manual or electrically powered chair) with one companion. There would be insufficient space for most wheelchairs to turn around.
Type 3 - BSEN81-70: 2003 2000 mm width by 1400 mm depth opening door width min 1100 mm	A user of any type of wheelchair together with several other passengers. There would be sufficient space for users with wheelchair and other mobility aids to turn a full circle.

Lift cars smaller than 1100 mm × 1400 mm may still accommodate a wheelchair user, but not one who requires assistance. In determining if an existing small lift is useable, the position of lift controls and safety features is critical.

Minimum car dimensions are measured between the structural walls of the car. Finishes must not encroach into these dimensions by more than 15 mm (total). Handrails and other fittings must be positioned so that they do not reduce manoeuvring space.

See 6.3.3

12.6 Platform lifts

The difference between installing a lifting platform and a wheelchair platform lift in an existing building is that a lifting platform requires a vertical lift shaft for its operation and a wheelchair platform lift operates and runs at an angle up the string of an existing staircase.

See 12.7

12.6.1 Platform lift requirements

Platform lifts should:

Visibility

- have the location of the lift within the sight of a member of staff where possible
- have doors which are clearly distinguishable from the adjoining walls
- have areas of glass which are clearly identifiable by people with a visual impairment.

Ease of approach

- provide adequate space for approach by wheelchair users.

Usability

- have suitable controls, gates and barriers for independent use by wheelchair users
- be designed to meet the needs of both ambulant disabled people and wheelchair users
- be designed to take both manual and most electric wheelchairs.

Good communication

- have clear operating instructions that can be read by a wheelchair user
- provide audible and visual announcements of platform level and floor reached
- minimise the use of visually and acoustically reflective wall surfaces.

Safety of use

- conform to the relevant British Standard EN 81 series of standards
- have a rated speed not exceeding 0.15 m/sec
- be fitted with continuous pressure controls, for example a push button or joystick
- be used with appropriate staff trained to assist people when using the lift
- have procedures in place to prevent unauthorised use of the lift.

12.6.2 Minimum dimensions

Platform lifts

Clear dimensions

The minimum clear dimensions of a platform lift are:

- 800 mm width × 1250 mm depth (unenclosed platform with provision for an unaccompanied wheelchair user) [Part M]
- 900 mm width × 1400 mm depth (enclosed platform with provision for an unaccompanied wheelchair) [Part M]
- 1100 mm width × 1400 mm depth (where two doors are located at 90° relative to each other and where the platform is enclosed, or where there is provision for an unaccompanied wheelchair user) [Part M].

Doors

- doors to lifting platforms should have a clear minimum effective width of 900 mm (for an 1100 mm width by 1400 mm depth platform) and a clear minimum effective width of 800 mm in all other cases.

Controls

- controls for lifting platforms should be located between 800 mm and 1100 mm affl and a minimum of 400 mm from any return wall
- controls for landings should be located between 900 mm and 1100 mm affl and a minimum of 500 mm from any return wall.

12.6.3 Travel distances

The travel distances for lifting platforms are:

- 2 metres maximum where there is no liftway enclosure and no floor penetration
- greater than 2 metres where there is a liftway enclosure.

The travel distance for a wheelchair platform lift will be determined by the flight rise of the stairs on which it is installed.

12.6.4 Aesthetics

The design of a platform lift can be adapted to fit sympathetically within the existing building, by matching it with the materials used in the original construction. Good design will result in a platform lift that fits seamlessly into its surroundings.

12.6.5 Space

If there is limited space within the existing building for installation of a platform lift, it may be necessary to create additional space by moving existing internal walls. Care must be taken to ensure that the structural stability of the building is not affected. However, there may be consequences of carrying out this type of work, including reduced room sizes, narrow corridors, and irregularly shaped accommodation.

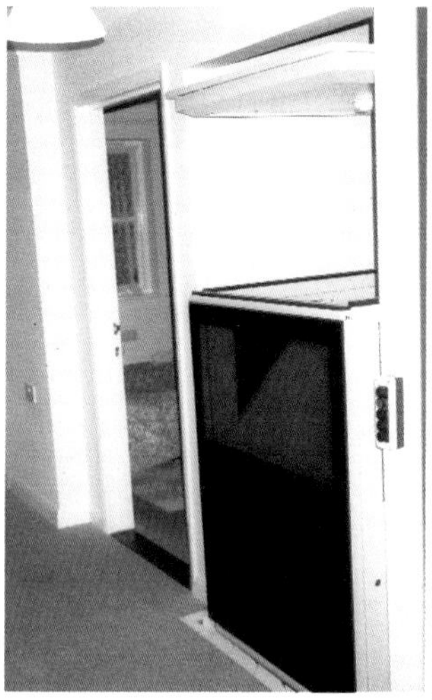

8. A platform lift fitted in a large residential accommodation.

12.6.6 Use

Platform lifts have some disadvantages when compared with a ramp or passenger lift. Their presence represents a provision for use only by disabled people and shows that other forms of vertical travel in the building are inaccessible to them. They also separate disabled people from others using the building and independence is reduced, as disabled users will need assistance in using them.

12.6.7 Space for future provision

If the improvement budget will not cover the cost of the lift installation, it may be possible to provide space and electrical supply as part of a refurbishment. This will allow the lift to be installed with reduced disruption when money becomes available.

12.7 Platform stairlifts and domestic stairlifts

12.7.1 Types of stairlift

There are two kinds of stairlifts, a domestic stairlift and a platform stairlift. A domestic stairlift incorporates a small platform and a seat, and is suitable only for people who can walk but experience difficulty climbing stairs. A platform stairlift is suitable for wheelchair users.

For existing buildings, it is important to consult a lift manufacturer at the earliest opportunity to discuss the type and requirements of the most suitable stairlift to be installed. Stairlifts should be used as a last resort because they are primarily intended for use in residential buildings and have a limited use.

See 6.3.3

12.7.2 Stairlift requirements

Stairlifts should:

- be used only when it is not possible to install a conventional passenger or platform lift
- conform to the requirements of BS 5776: 1996 *Specification for Powered Stairlifts*
- only be installed in a building with two or more staircases, on the staircase that is not intended for use as a means of escape
- only be installed in a building with a single staircase when a clear stairway width can be maintained between the carriage rail of the stairlift and the handrail opposite.

Usability

- should be easy to operate with clear instructions
- have minimum clear dimensions for a wheelchair platform lift of:
  - 1050 mm width by 1250 mm depth [BS 8300: 2001]
  - 800 mm width by 1250 mm depth [Part M]
- doors for wheelchair platform lifts should have a minimum effective width of 800 mm.

Safety of use

- be located within sight of a member of staff who can assist users in case of difficulty
- be fitted with an alarm that conforms to the requirements of ISO 9386-2
- have controls that are designed to prevent unauthorised use (ISO 9386-2)
- not obstruct the required clear width of a staircase when parked.

12.7.3 Limited use

The advantages of a platform stairlift over a passenger lift are that its installation does not require a pit and it usually causes less noise and disturbance than with the installation of a passenger lift. In existing buildings, a platform stairlift is less expensive to install; the disadvantage is that there may be a limit in the vertical distance that can be travelled. A platform stairlift should be installed in an existing building only when it is not practical to install a platform lift or passenger lift.

12.7.4 Means of escape and stairlifts

For means of escape in case of an emergency refer to Chapter 15 Evacuation.

See 3.4.3, 3.8, 3.9, 15.1, 15.4

12.8 Escalators and passenger conveyors

Escalator and passenger conveyors should conform to BS EN 115.

Generally, they should:

Good communication

- incorporate clear signage directing users to an alternative lift or staircase
- incorporate clear signage identifying the location of the escalator or passenger conveyor and the direction of travel
- have handrails which contrast in colour and luminance when viewed against their background.

Safety of use

- incorporate guarding along each side and at each end of the conveyor as a safety precaution, particularly for people with a visual impairment.

Conveyors, sometimes used instead of escalators, can be too steep for wheelchairs, presenting a danger of the wheelchair tipping backwards or forwards, and loss of control by the user.

Signage should clearly indicate the gradient of the conveyor and management policies should ensure assistance is available if required.

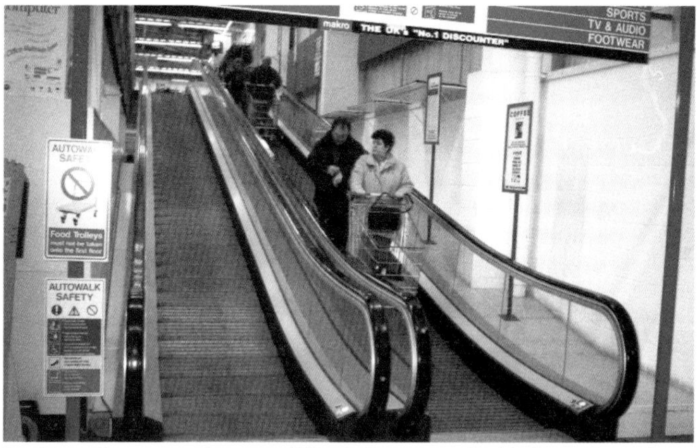

9. Travellators can be very difficult for many disabled people and impossible, and very dangerous, for others. Wheelchair users can tip backwards when ascending or lose control when descending.

See 4.3.4, 14.2.1

12.9 Lighting

Good lighting is essential for safety on stairs and when using facilities such as passenger, platform and stair lifts. Good practice guidance for lighting is given in Chapter 13.

13 Lighting, colour and acoustics

Colour, lighting and acoustics play an important part in assisting all users to enjoy an environment, and this is especially so for disabled people.

As well as affecting the general visual appearance of an environment, colour and luminance, contrast can be used to highlight features that assist disabled people to move around independently and safely. Lighting also plays a major role in the aesthetic appeal of an environment and in judging its accessibility to disabled people. Appropriate lighting, with respect to design, installation and maintenance, is essential. The acoustics of an environment can also influence its usability. For some disabled people, poor acoustics can hinder, or even prevent, communication. This chapter considers these three important aspects of accessibility.

13.1 Design principles – lighting

It may be necessary to change, reposition and/or supplement the lighting to enhance the use of an environment by disabled people. There may also be a need to change the type of lighting, the luminaires, lamps or controls, or to reposition switches and change the type of switch and/or the colour. Improvements will often benefit many users of a building and this may strengthen the case for using money allocated for general improvements, to improve the appearance and safety of the building.

Replacement of luminaires can be made at little, or no extra cost if they are undertaken as part of a refurbishment or maintenance programme, or as work undertaken in response to a schedule of dilapidations at the end of a lease, or because of changes in legislation.

A glossary of lighting terminology is provided in section 13.1.6.

13.1.1 Basic principles of good lighting to ensure accessibility

The amount of natural and artificial lighting available within an environment should suit the tasks to be performed and the abilities of individual users. In general:

- good lighting should meet all the health and safety requirements of the space
- lighting should provide sufficient illuminance to allow for tasks to be carried out and for the main features within a space to be identified
- light reflected from ceilings, walls or floors increases the light flowing within a room and helps to produce a more uniform distribution of light. This, in turn, will reduce dark areas and strong shadows.
- lighting should have a low Glare Index and avoid the incidence of "Disability Glare" (see glossary)
- good general lighting should be provided with higher illuminance at potential hazards (for example, steps and ramps) and where good visibility is required (for example, signs, controls, workstations, reception counters)

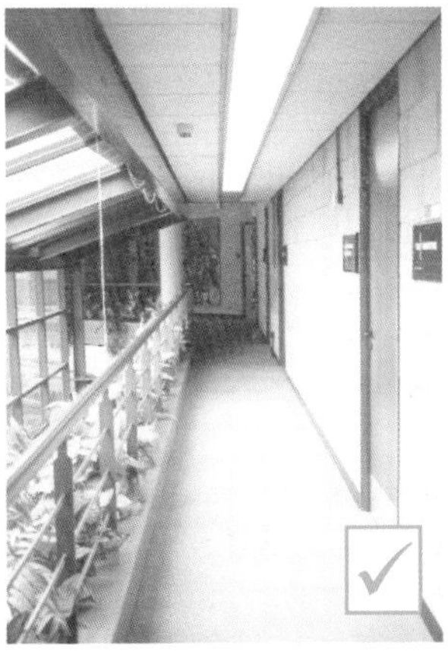

1. Good example of evenly distributed lighting in a complicated environment.

- the direction of lighting should not cause glare or confusing shadows. In workplaces, the main artificial lighting should be diffused and, if possible, reflected off light surfaces such as ceilings. Daylight and sunlight should be controllable by curtains or blinds.
- a directional component to lighting helps to accentuate facial modelling which is useful in lip reading and the use of sign language. It can also highlight the position of signs, doors and notice boards, and create contrasting shadows that make the shapes, such as stair treads and risers, more visible.
- lighting controls should be positioned so they are accessible to wheelchair users. They should be easy to operate and allow occupants to control the lighting in the part of the space they are using.

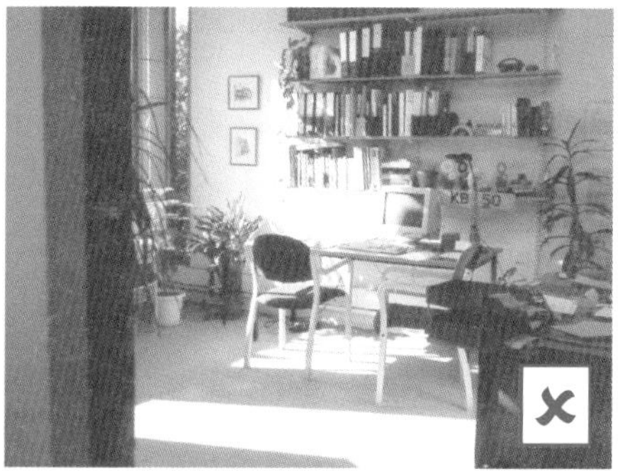

2. The confusing shadows on the floor of this office may cause problems for visually impaired people.

- the lighting provided should meet the colour appearance and colour rendering requirements of the space
- colour and luminance contrast may be lost when some types of lamps are used
- the illuminance immediately inside and outside entrances should allow for adaptation of vision when entering or leaving a building. Adapting to a change in illuminance can take much longer for users with a visual impairment. Gradual changes in lighting immediately inside and outside the entrance of a building (especially at night) should be sufficient to allow visual adaptation.
- lighting at reception counters or other communication points should be designed to enhance facial modelling, making lip reading easier
- circulation routes should be uniformly lit, avoiding glare and strong shadows
- lighting must be well maintained
- glare should be avoided as it can lead to accidents and collisions, for example, if there is a brightly lit, uncurtained window at the head of a stair or at the end of a corridor
- the level of emergency lighting should allow for the needs of users with visual impairments.

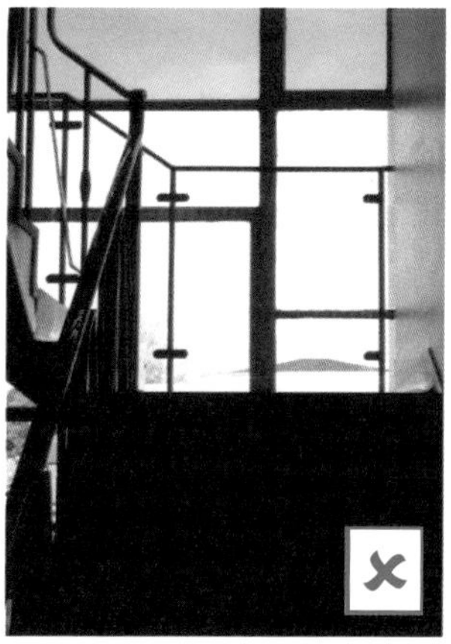

3. The uncurtained window at the top of this staircase can cause glare and confusing shadows on the staircase, particularly on a bright sunny day. The use of a window blind which can be adjusted depending upon the amount of daylight entering the staircase will help to minimise the problem.

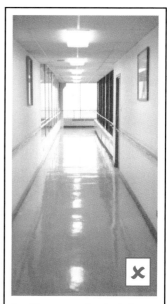

4. The uncurtained window at the end of this corridor and the position of the overhead lighting have caused glare and confusing shadows on the floor of the corridor.

See 13.1.2

More than 95 per cent of people with a visual impairment have some perception of light and dark. Good quality lighting will not only help them to maximise their residual vision but will also improve conditions for all other users of the environment.

While increasing the illuminance may not actually be helpful for some people with visual impairments, providing the ability to control both the amount of illuminance and the direction of the light will assist in meeting the needs of most people.

The ceiling is usually an unobstructed area, so people with visual impairments will look for contrast at the wall/ceiling junction to assess the size and shape of the room they have entered. This is a more difficult task where the ceiling is poorly lit. Ceiling-mounted luminaires can directly illuminate the ceiling, whereas luminaires that are recessed into the ceiling (commonly installed to control veiling reflections in computer screens) can provide dark ceilings.

Daylight may provide all or only some of the lighting for a building during the day, with artificial lighting being used at night. For environments that operate during both day and night, such as transport environments, or those that will be used during darker days in winter, such as offices, shops etc, it is essential that the relationship between the lighting and, for example, manifestation on glass and colour contrast or signage, is effective in both lighting regimes.

Light sources positioned above the centre line of a circulation route, will enhance visual clues along a route. Deep shadows and abrupt changes in lighting levels from one space to another must be avoided, but soft shadows can add form to the visual image for people with visual impairments, helping them locate and identify features within a building. However, creating soft shadows must be carried out with care.

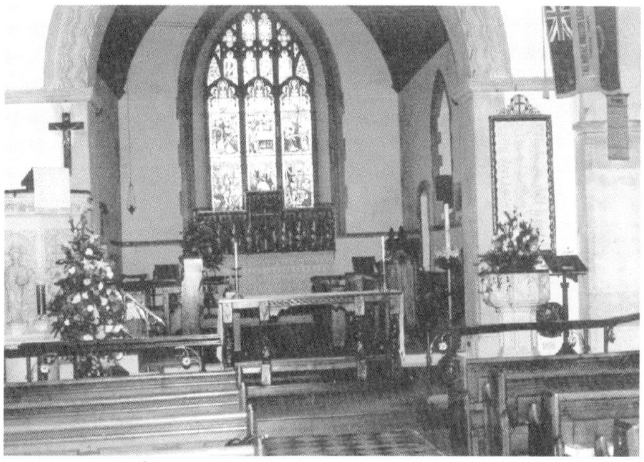

5. It is not only offices and shops that operate during the day and at night. In this church it may be difficult for hearing impaired people to lip read when a sermon is being given because of the amount of glare through the stained glass window at certain times of the day.

13.1.2 Sources of light in an environment

Artificial light

Typically, this is produced electrically and gives an almost constant illuminance. The further away surfaces are from the luminaire, the less light they will receive. Light flows in a three dimensional way and can reveal the structure and form of the building. This flow of light can help to identify features and occupants, so that the building may operate as an inclusive and accessible environment.

Natural light or daylight

Natural light, or daylight, is a variable source but is still considered by many to be the ideal light source. The sky, even when overcast, can provide a good amount of useful light. However, the orientation of windows and roof lights is critical for optimising daylight.

Artificial lighting design – key features

The designer of artificial lighting needs to consider the following issues in order to produce an effective design solution:

- artificial lighting design assumes that there is no natural daylight available
- the selection of suitable luminaires, with their associated light sources, will involve both engineering design and judgements on aesthetics
- the colour temperature and colour rendering of the light source are critical for the colour appearance of the space
- the number and position of the luminaires will influence the appearance of the interior and/or exterior space as well as the amount of light that is falling on surfaces and flowing around the space
- luminaires are commonly the brightest source of light in the visual field and are frequently a source of glare
- the veiling reflections of luminaires in computer screens can cause disability glare, making it impossible to see images and text on the screen
- to provide the required maintained illuminance in a space, cleaning fittings, re-lamping luminaires and re-decoration of interior surfaces is critical. An accessible environment may be lost simply because of poor maintenance.
- the random replacement of lamps of a different type from those used in the original design, can be detrimental to the colour appearance of the space

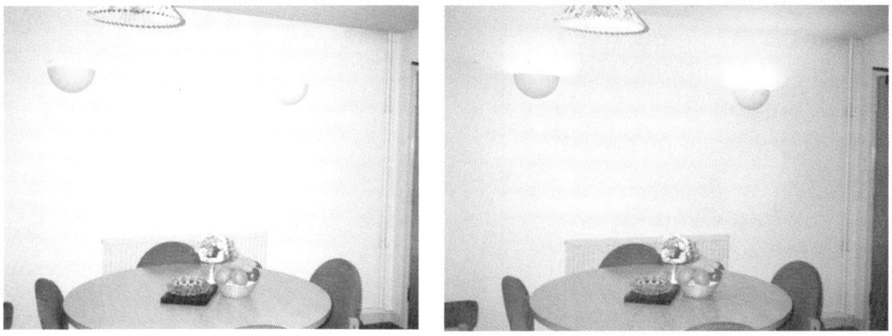

6 & 7. The source of lighting can produce differing effects within an environment.

- lighting design computer programs are available to provide approximate visualisations of interior spaces when they are lit
- artificial lighting can be controlled in a number of ways. Wherever possible, controls that allow variations should be included, such as dimmer switches controlling small groups of luminaires. These controls are now available for smooth dimming of fluorescent lamps.

For further information on the design of artificial lighting, several texts are available (Society of Light and Lighting, 2001; Tregenza and Loe, 1998; Cuttel, 2003).

Natural lighting or daylighting design – key features

The dynamic nature and the unique colour rendering of natural light can give a special quality to interior spaces.

The amount of useful light that is produced from the sky and flows into buildings is not usually defined as "illuminance" and the traditional method for design has been to use the Daylight Factor approach. The position of the sun can be used to make predictions of sunlight penetration into buildings.

The sun can cause considerable glare for occupants, especially through south facing windows. A range of shading devices is available to control this.

As with artificial lighting, there are computer programs that provide approximate visualisations of the interior spaces lit by daylight.

The following issues should be addressed in producing an effective design solution:

- natural lighting design of interior spaces often includes a contribution from artificial lighting
- natural light is dynamic, giving changing lighting patterns
- the selection of the shape and position of windows, roof lights, and shading devices will fundamentally affect the lighting and appearance of the space
- the nature of daylight makes it difficult to match exactly with artificial light sources
- windows and roof lights, as the brightest source of light in the visual field, are frequently a source of glare
- sunlight on shiny surfaces can produce veiling reflections causing disability glare
- failure to clean and maintain the glass and glazing will result in a reduction of the natural lighting being transmitted through the glass
- natural light can produce strong shadows that can be disorientating for users
- natural lighting design computer programs are available to provide approximate visualisations of interior spaces when they are lit
- natural lighting can be controlled in a number of ways. Blinds, curtains and shutters offer some control. External louvres and shelves can be used to reduce the amount of direct sunlight entering the room and to reflect natural light off the ceiling in a more diffuse manner.

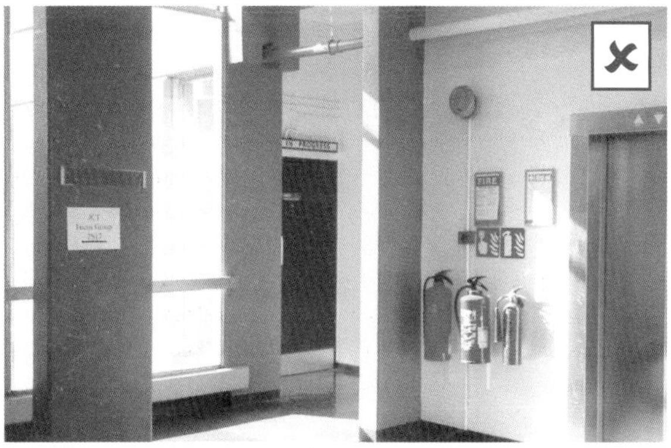

8. The changes in natural lighting coming into a building can be dramatic, and very visually confusing for all users.

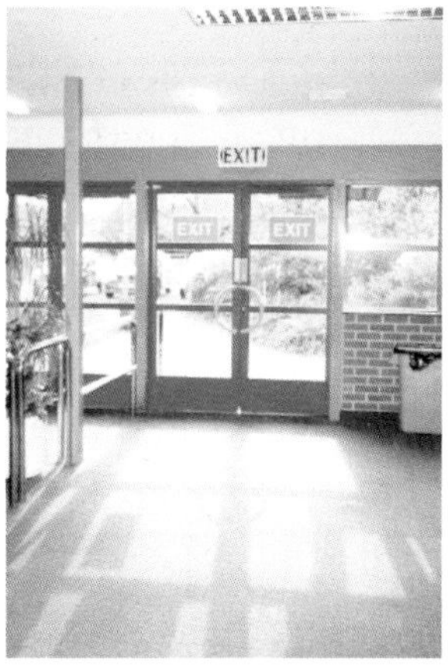

9. Some control of the light entering the building and producing shadows at floor level would be useful here.

For further information on the design of natural lighting or daylighting, a range of texts is available. (BSI, 1985; Tregenza and Loe, 1998; Ander, 2003)

13.1.3 Task lighting

Some people with a visual impairment require higher illuminance when undertaking tasks but, for some, too much light can cause discomfort, pain and disorientation. Some light sources also generate heat, which can be dangerous for someone who needs to work close to the lamp.

It is essential that people with visual impairments are allowed to control the lighting for their tasks and at their workstations. Task lighting should be selected only when the specific needs of a visually impaired user are known and properly assessed.

The general lighting of the space should also be sufficient to minimise adaptation problems that may occur as people move from task to general lighting.

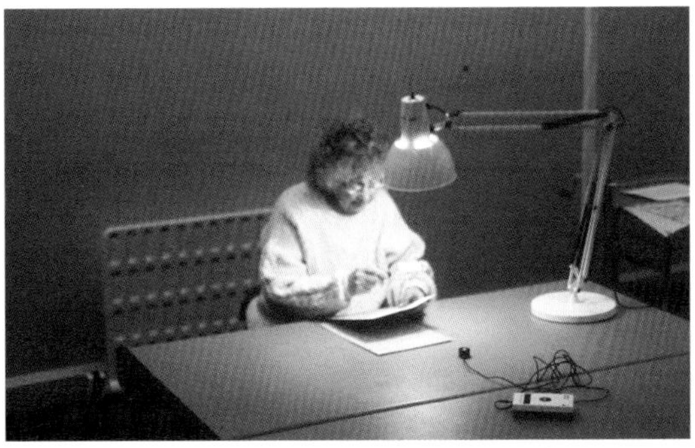

10 & 11. The type of task lamp provided should meet the individual needs of the user.

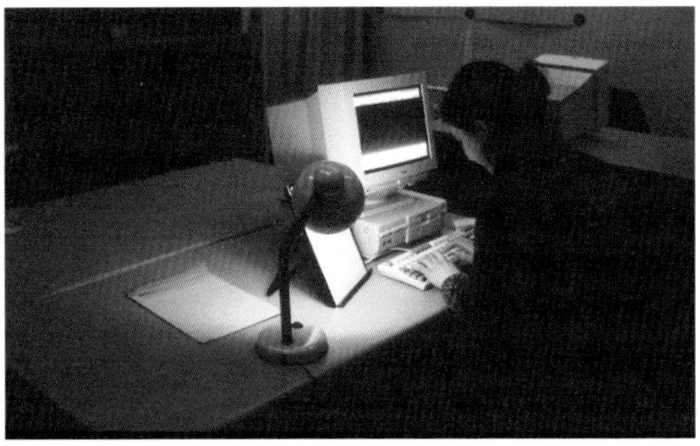

See 14.2.2

13.1.4 Lighting controls

In most cases, different illuminance is needed for different tasks. The varying needs of users, in terms of the amount of light they actually need or would prefer, means flexibility of control is essential. Providing a simple on/off option on a single switch to an area should always be avoided.

In general, lighting can also be controlled by:

- dimmer switches – now available for fluorescent lamps
- pull cords
- push plates that move through a cycle of settings allowing one to be selected when pressure is released
- infrared and other remote control devices
- presence detectors
- intelligent luminaires that "learn" to adjust their output to provide a uniform illuminance for the task.

Controls should never require the simultaneous use of both hands.

In areas where pull cords are also provided for security calls or to operate emergency systems, such as in an accessible toilet, it is essential that pull cords are appropriately identified by colour: red for alarms and white for lighting control.

Details of the positioning of controls are given in Chapter 14.

See 13.1.1

13.1.5 Recommended illuminance

Table 13a Illuminance recommendations (source BS8300: 2001)

Location	Illuminance	Comment
Ramps	100	min at top and bottom of ramp
External steps	100	min at tread level
Entrance	200*	SMI at floor level
Corridor	100*	SMI at floor level
Internal stairs	100	min at tread level
Internal ramps	100	min at top and bottom of ramp
Lavatory	100	SMI at floor level
Bathroom	100 to 300	SMI at sink level
Shower area	100 to 300	SMI at sink level
Bedroom	100	min at floor level
Kitchen	150 to 300	SMI at worktop level

Notes:
* = Illuminance recommendations taken from the SSL Code for Lighting 2001
min = minimum illuminance
SMI = Standard Maintained Illuminance (lux).

See 9.4.6, 13.1.1, 13.1.2, 13.1.6

13.1.6 Lighting – a glossary of terms

There are a number of terms used in lighting, which include the following:

Illuminance

The amount of light falling on a surface, measured in Lumens/square metre (lm/m^2). This is also called "lux".

Standard maintained illuminance

The minimum lux provided for a specific interior, even allowing for the depreciation of the lighting regime due to normal use. The maintained illuminance of the interior would occur just before the lighting regime undergoes maintenance and should be provided on the surface where the tasks are to be carried out. For kitchens, this may be at worktop level; for external and emergency lighting, it may be at ground or floor level.

Luminance

The amount of light either reflected or emitted from a surface, measured in candelas/square metre (cd/m^2). Typically, this is assumed to be the light on a horizontal surface, but vertical illuminance is also important, particularly for external lighting and for modelling people or objects within the space.

Colour rendering index

The colour performance of a lamp is described by its colour rendering index. This is the ability to show colours accurately. A value of 100 is considered excellent (CIE, 1988).

Colour temperature

This describes the light from a lamp which determines its appearance in terms of warmth or coolness.

Daylight factor

The ratio of the total amount of natural lighting or daylight from the sky to the amount of natural lighting or daylight that is present at a position in a room within a building. This is expressed as a percentage (%).

Diversity

The ratio of minimum to maximum illuminance across a specified room or space.

Uniformity

The ratio of minimum illuminance to the average illuminance across a specified room or space.

Adaptation

The process that takes place as a person's vision adjusts itself to the brightness or colour of the visual scene. This may take several seconds or minutes for people with a visual impairment.

Light sources

There are two main types of light sources available:

- incandescent lamps
- discharge lamps.

The first group includes normal light bulbs and tungsten halogen lamps that start instantly and provide reasonable colour rendering. They can be very bright and cause glare if not used carefully. Tungsten halogen lamps are commonly used as spotlights. Incandescent lamps are generally described as having a "warm" colour temperature.

The most common discharge lamp is the fluorescent lamp which, like all types of discharge lamp, requires time to achieve full light output after being switched on. Fluorescent lamps are commonly described as having a "cool" colour temperature. The use of electronic controls with fluorescent lamps can overcome the interference sometimes caused to hearing aids by this type of lamp.

Lamps can also be differentiated by their colour rendering performance. There are a large number of different lamps and further information can be obtained from the Lighting Industry Federation (LIF, 2003)

Luminaires

These are more commonly called lighting fittings. There are a great variety of luminaires available and manufacturers provide technical and appearance information in a standard format for use by lighting designers. An important function of a luminaire is to direct light from the lamp to where it is required in a safe and efficient manner. Task lights are specialised types of luminaire.

Discomfort glare

This is defined by reference to a Glare Index (CIBSE, 1985) which takes into account the position of the glare sources relative to the viewing direction, and its brightness (or luminance). Interiors with a Glare Index >20 are likely to be "glarey".

As the Glare Index is attributable to all of the lighting in a room, the index for specific viewing directions may also need to be determined.

Disability glare

This can occur in building interiors when shiny surfaces are illuminated. The resulting reflections, which produce bright patches of light, can mask the nature of the reflecting surface. These so called "veiling reflections" cause disability glare with respect to the reflecting surface.

A range of definitions are included in the Society of Light and Lighting (SLL), The lighting code (SLL, 2001) Note: BS 8206 Part 1, Code of practice for artificial lighting, has been superseded by the SLL Code for lighting 2001.

13.2 Colour

13.2.1 The role of colour in an accessible environment

In an existing building, colour and luminance contrast can help disabled people to move around, identify features and communicate with others. Redecoration will probably take place several times throughout the life of a building, giving many opportunities to improve accessibility. The appropriate selection and use of colours can do this – all at no additional cost. Unfortunately, the poor use of colour brought about by a lack of understanding of best practice can also seriously hinder accessibility.

Colour and luminance contrast of major surface areas such as walls, floors and ceilings will assist disabled people in moving around a building. On handrails, architraves, skirting boards, doors and controls (for example light switches, sockets etc), it can greatly enhance the ability of a disabled person to identify and use important facilities and safety features.

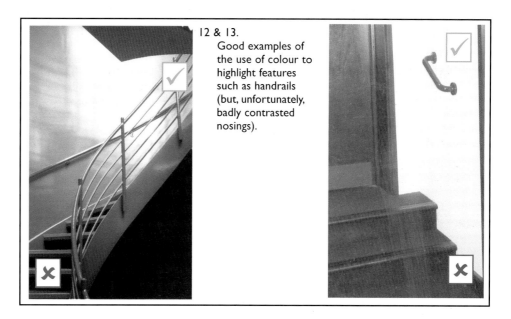

12 & 13.
Good examples of the use of colour to highlight features such as handrails (but, unfortunately, badly contrasted nosings).

The effectiveness of colour and luminance contrast in an interior space is strongly influenced by the lighting regime and this should be fully integrated within the design process.

13.2.2 Specific requirements for people with visual impairments

Visual impairment can cause a large number of different effects on colour vision. People with a particular impairment may not see certain colours very well, and their ability to see colours may change with time.

People with visual impairments may detect a colour by:

- its intensity
- its ability to reflect light
- a combination of the above.

A reliance on selecting colours from different parts of the spectrum (a different hue), is less effective than making a selection based on the colour and luminance contrast, as some people are unable to detect differences in hue.

It is the relative brightness of the surface or the illuminance that is important in providing a coloured environment. The difference in luminance between two adjacent surfaces is termed the luminance contrast. Different colours can provide an acceptable luminance contrast but some colours under similar lighting conditions can appear to have equal luminance.

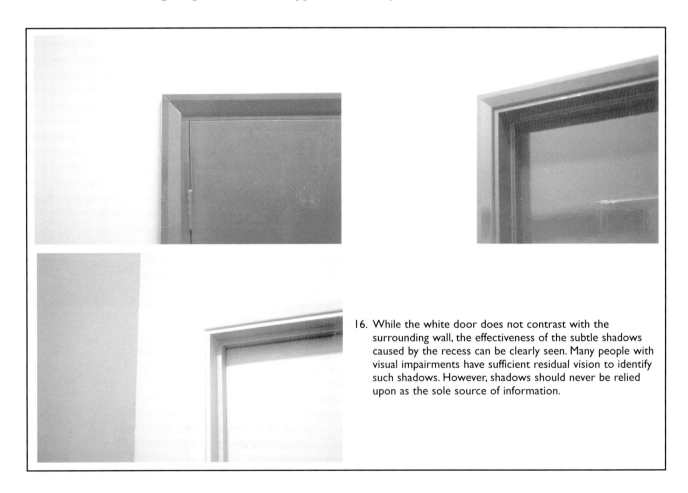

16. While the white door does not contrast with the surrounding wall, the effectiveness of the subtle shadows caused by the recess can be clearly seen. Many people with visual impairments have sufficient residual vision to identify such shadows. However, shadows should never be relied upon as the sole source of information.

In this case there will be no luminance contrast. Design guidance is now available to enable the selection of colours for an interior so that adequate luminance contrast is provided to meet the meets of most people with visual impairments. (Bright *et al*, 1997).

13.2.3 The influence of reflection and position of surfaces

Although many surfaces in buildings have a matt finish, those that are shiny generate reflections and cause glare, which can be confusing for people with visual impairments. The ability of deaf people and people with hearing impairments to lip read can also be more difficult in environments where there is glare and reflection.

Large mirrors, open areas of glass and shiny metal surfaces, can be particularly problematic.

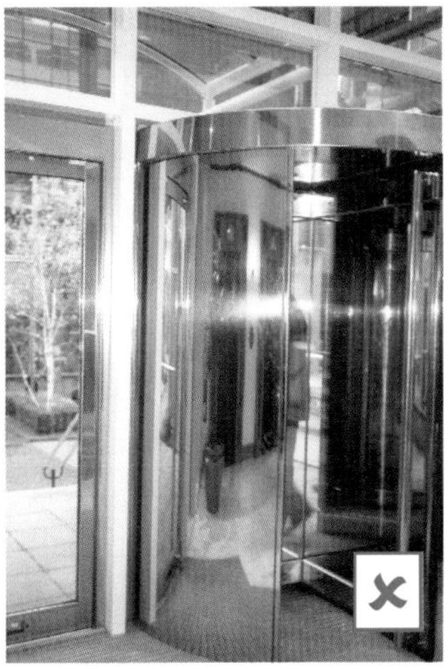

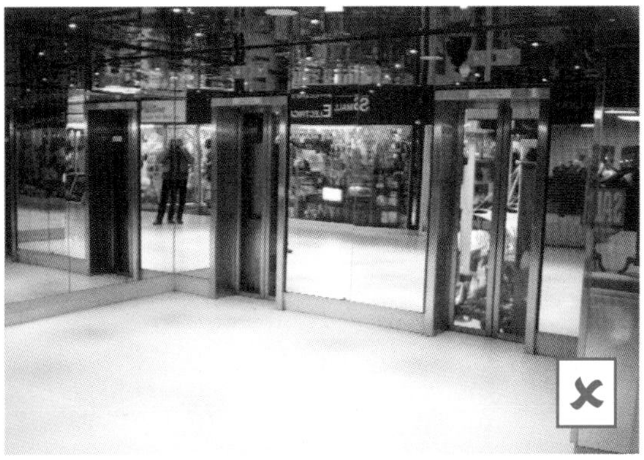

17 &18 Mirrored and shiny surfaces can cause problems when navigating around a building.

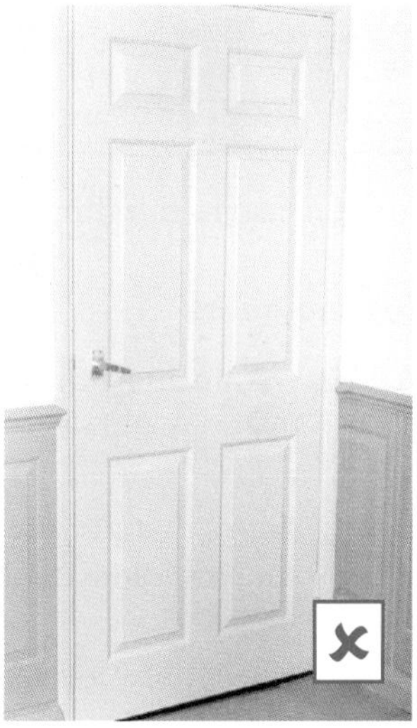

19. The lack of colour contrast between the wall and the floor makes this room appear larger than it is for people with vision problems. They think that the edge of the room is where the contrast is more obvious – the junction of the dado rail with the wall.

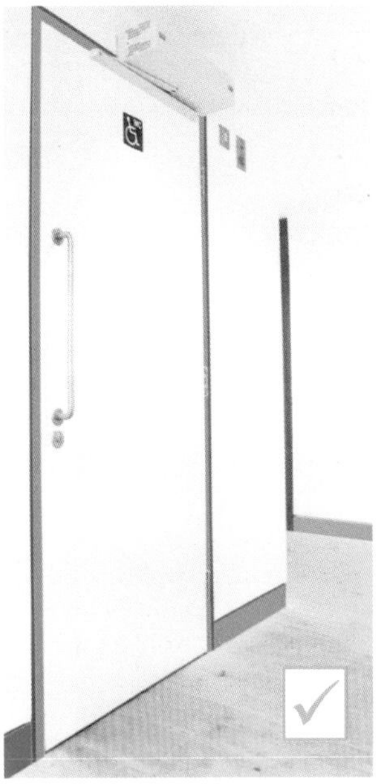

20. In this example, the good colour contrast between the skirting board and the floor makes the edges of the door and corridor clearly distinguishable and easy to identify.

On entering a room, people with a visual impairment will usually pause and try to gather information about the space they have just entered. Contrast at the junction of the wall and ceiling, which is often the least cluttered area in the space, can be particularly helpful. However, when moving around, people with visual impairments rarely look at the ceiling but rather concentrate their vision within 2 m in front of them, looking downwards and continually scanning the scene to about 1500 mm affl.

Contrast between the wall and the floor is critical as a source of information when moving around and, whilst contrast may be provided as a useful source of information at the ceiling/wall junction, it must be provided at the junction of the wall/floor to assist navigation.

All surfaces within the building should be considered as an integrated system that provides adequate luminance contrast and texture for people to use the building independently. Adequate luminance contrast will also reveal potential hazards.

13.2.4 Design overview

To provide an accessible environment:

- avoid floor, wall, door and ceiling surfaces of high gloss
- use luminance contrast to identify the junctions of floors, walls, doors and ceilings
- freestanding columns should contrast with the background walls
- architrave should provide adequate luminance contrast to the wall
- skirting should provide adequate luminance contrast to the floor
- use textured surfaces in floor finishes as hazard warnings
- floor surfaces need to be slip-resistant and provide a good wheel-grip
- avoid large repeating patterns with colours of high chroma
- consider using colour to identify one space, level or area from another.

Colours for use in buildings may be specified using British Standards (BSI, 1976; BSI, 1989)

Routes and doors

- colour and luminance contrast should be used to distinguish accessible routes and to distinguish between routes for particular purposes
- doors that are used for specific purposes (for example, maintenance) could be a similar colour to the adjacent wall
- doors used for access should be easily identifiable
- where doors are likely to be left open, the leading edge of the door should be made visible using good luminance contrast.

Distinguishing spaces

- identical spaces on circulation routes should be avoided
- colour, lighting and furnishings should be used to distinguish between spaces that may be confused with each other
- spaces that are usually easily distinguished by outlook and daylighting may not look the same after dark under artificial lighting
- at similar entrances, the arrangement of the reception desk and type of seating should be different.

13.2.5 Redecoration

Redecoration should take into account:

- the need to make light switches and other controls visible
- the higher background lighting levels that can be achieved with light wall and ceiling surfaces.

See 4.1.1, 4.7.6, 11.2.2, 13.2.1

13.3 Acoustics

13.3.1 Good acoustic environment

The acoustic environment is critical for all users, but especially for those users who are deaf or hard of hearing or who have a visual impairment. High levels of background noise will affect the ability of a person with a hearing impairment to distinguish speech, or to use any hearing they do have to gain details from audible information systems. Hearing aids amplify sound at the ear including that present in the general environment. This can make it difficult for a person who has a hearing impairment to engage in a conversation.

In any room or space containing a sound source, the amount of sound at any particular position is made up of two components:

1 The direct component is the amount of sound power in the sound source and the distance away from the source. Designing the source of the sound to be quieter is an option. Alternatively, increasing the distance from the sound source may reduce the sound to an acceptable level.

2. The reverberant component is the sound that has been reflected from surfaces within the room or space after leaving the sound source.

The reduction of severe background noise is beneficial but people with visual impairments often use reflected sound to gain information about the space they are in, or to hear if someone is approaching them.

For all users, a well-designed acoustic environment is beneficial. General guidance is available in BS 8233 (BSI, 1999b).

13.3.2 Design overview

To provide an accessible acoustic environment:

- the extensive use of hard materials that have low absorption coefficients should be avoided
- the advantages of absorbent floor finishes must be balanced with any problems that soft surfaces have on wheelchair accessibility
- materials and surfaces that are sound-absorbent should be used to provide an environment that is sufficiently reverberant to provide some acoustic liveliness
- the attenuation of loud sound sources should be considered. Building services with moving parts are commonly a source of high sound levels.
- the frequency range of the general sound in the space should be identified, since high frequency sounds may be quiet but still annoying.

The design guidance produced by CIBSE, 2002, Guide B5: *Noise and Vibration Control for HVCA*, ISBN: 1 903287 25 1 (CIBSE, 2002), provides additional information concerning the acoustic properties of spaces and rooms.

13.3.3 Sound-absorbent finishes

The ability of people to follow a conversation can be affected by the level of ambient sound and its characteristics (ie continuous low pitch is less of a problem than intermittent sounds of a higher pitch). For people with a hearing impairment, the adverse effect of high ambient sound levels is exaggerated.

An environment with low levels of background noise is critical for people with hearing impairments. When the background noise level is high, people shout to be heard and the general noise level increases.

Hard finishes reflect sound and the effect can be a noisy environment that makes it particularly difficult for a person with a hearing impairment to understand what is being said. This is termed a reverberant room or space.

Sound absorbance

Sound-absorbent materials on ceilings, walls, floors and furnishings, prevent some of the sound being reflected. The ability of a surface to absorb sound is quantified by the absorption coefficient. A high absorption coefficient means that much of the sound is absorbed. Carpets and furniture fabrics have high coefficients. Floor tiles and metal have low absorption coefficients.

Affecting sound absorbance

In any interior there will be a variety of different materials and surfaces and each will have a different absorption coefficient. The overall effect of these surfaces can be quantified to produce an accessible acoustic environment.

Reverberation time is important for people with a hearing impairment. This is the time taken for a loud noise to decay. Interiors with high reverberation times are more difficult for people with hearing impairments as there is reverberant background sound masking what they are attempting to hear. These places are acoustically "live".

Rooms having low sound-absorption materials will have long reverberation times. Conversely, rooms or spaces with high sound-absorption materials will have short reverberation times. This can produce spaces or rooms that are acoustically "dead".

Soft or resilient floor finishes can be used to reduce the sound of footsteps but this must be balanced with the need for firm surfaces for easy operation of wheelchairs. Deep piled carpets, for example, are very difficult and tiring for a wheelchair user to negotiate, especially but not exclusively, over long distances.

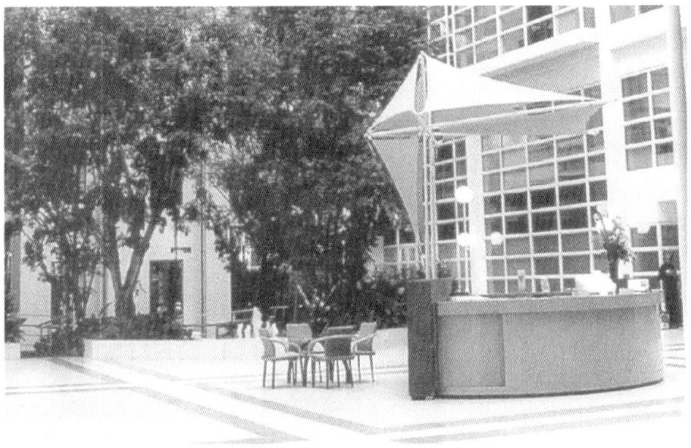

21. Acoustic cover over a reception desk in a large, acoustically "live" environment

13.3.4 Pitch and frequency of sound

The pitch or frequency of a sound is also important. In general, the ear is more sensitive to high frequencies and even some fairly quiet high frequency sounds can be annoying and distracting for people with sensory impairments. Low frequency sounds are less of a problem. To create an accessible acoustic environment it must be remembered that the sound absorption characteristics of materials and surfaces change with frequency.

13.3.5 Sound attenuation

Sources of ambient sound should be controlled or masked. Sound attenuation techniques should be used to reduce ambient noise from equipment, perhaps involving acoustic linings or covers.

Fans and pumps can be set on resilient mountings and enclosed. It may be possible to shield reception counters from telephone bells, public address announcements and adjacent conversations.

14 Services

The services available within an environment are very important to disabled people in both the provision of the services and in how they are maintained. For many disabled people, how they are able to access and operate the equipment often associated with services is a critical factor in determining the usability of an environment.

14.1 Design principles

14.1.1 Comfortable conditions

Services should create comfortable conditions for all users of an existing building, but the internal environment is more critical for some disabled people than for non-disabled users. Lighting, background noise, water quality, water temperature, radiator temperature, air quality and air temperature, all have the potential to create discomfort and safety hazards for disabled people.

14.1.2 Ease of use and control

Ease of operation, visibility and height, are the key factors that affect the ease with which disabled people can use services. Operating services for all appliances and equipment are made easier if controls:

- require only a small amount of force to use
- are of a shape and size that is easy to grasp or to operate by a simple movement (eg push plate) and take into account the needs of people with limited dexterity
- are designed so that any controls that need to be used by disabled people do not require the simultaneous use of both hands
- are reachable by all users or, where appropriate, automatic
- have settings (eg on/off, high/low) that are easy to see
- have settings that can be determined audibly or by touch
- have operating instructions that are easily visible, are in simple language or have pictograms that are easy to understand, and with any associated information being of appropriate size and embossed
- are positioned consistently within a building
- do not need the user to climb or reach excessively in order to operate them (for example when opening a window positioned over a sink or wash hand basin, or to change fuses or read meters)
- use circuit breakers, rather than re-wirable fuses. These are easier to reset, especially by disabled people
- are contrasted in terms of colour and luminance with their background
- are not provided with the switches coloured red and green to denote off or on, as this may cause confusion for some users with a visual impairment or a colour identification deficit.

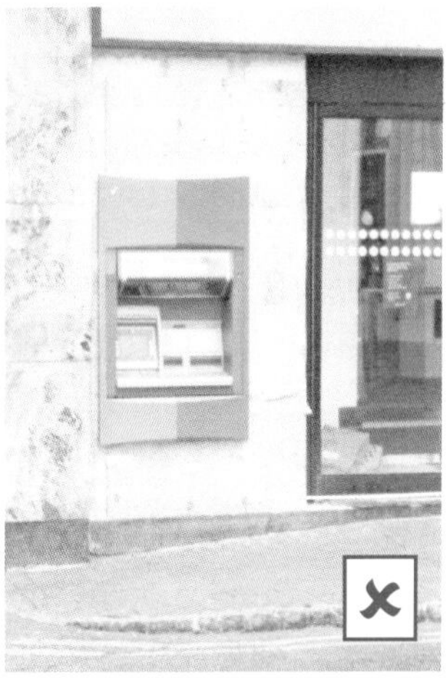

1. This ATM is easy to locate by using good colour contrast between the machine and the background against which it is viewed. However, the narrow sloping pavement would be a problem for wheelchair users.

14.2 Strategy for existing buildings

14.2.1 Existing services and controls

Any access audit of an existing building should include consideration of the services. Risk assessments in relation to health and safety policies will also include the building services and environment. Many similar issues will need to be addressed in assessing accessibility and risk (for example, air quality, temperature and lighting control for different tasks, water temperature due to risk of scalding). However, the measures needed to meet the requirements of disabled people may go further than those necessary to ensure the health and safety of non-disabled people.

A strategy must be developed to ensure that, when improvements to services are carried out, health and safety assessments reflect the needs of disabled people. Budgets for improvements to meet these needs should not have to cover general health and safety measures.

14.2.2 Services for use by staff

As many services are controlled by staff, specific improvements can be made to meet the needs of disabled users. For example, lights can be switched on and off by infrared or ultrasonic remote controls, and a telephone designed to suit the particular needs of people with hearing impairments can be connected at the desk where it is required. Task lighting should also be determined according to the particular needs of a disabled person.

14.2.3 Management

In terms of employment, the services made available to a disabled employee should be decided only after an independent workplace assessment of their needs has been carried out. General improvements in accessibility should always be made during routine maintenance and refurbishment. However, it is not possible to prejudge all the particular needs of a disabled member of staff, and some adjustments may be needed in each particular case. Funding should always be available for such eventualities, and management practices should be introduced to ensure that the needs of the employee are addressed as swiftly as possible. Access to Work schemes are available for just these types of adjustments.

See 3.2.5

14.3 Telephones

14.3.1 Location

A public telephone should usually be provided in the arrival space, or in another suitable accessible space, in any building regularly used by the public. It should be in a quiet area and at a suitable height for use by someone in a wheelchair, and there should be enough space for a wheelchair user to manoeuvre close to the phone.

Dimensions, shelves, handrails, signs and seats for a public telephone suitable for use by wheelchair users or ambulant disabled people, are shown in Figure 14a.

The provision of sound-absorbent materials around the public telephone will reduce reflected sound. The position of any sound-reducing canopy must not make it difficult for either disabled or non-disabled people to use the phone comfortably, nor should they obstruct circulation space.

14.3.2 Convenient telephones

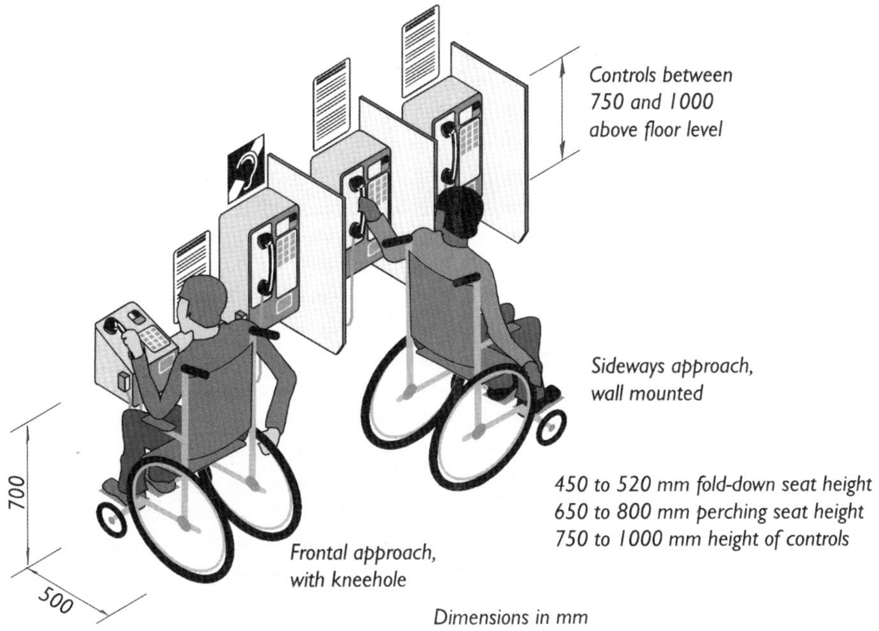

Figure 14a Public telephones for use by disabled people.

Telephones should be available, conveniently positioned and suitable for disabled people to use. Generally:

- public telephones should be available in buildings regularly visited by the public
- in buildings where public telephones are provided, at least one of the telephones should be reachable and visible from a wheelchair (if there is only one telephone, a seat, fold down if necessary, can be provided to make it usable by non-wheelchair users)
- there should be enough space in front of a public telephone to allow a wheelchair to approach it comfortably. Ideally, telephones for use by disabled people should be located to enable wheelchair users to approach and use the telephone from the front and the side. Where it is possible to approach a telephone only from the front, a knee recess at least 500 mm deep and 700 mm high, should be provided.
- if an opening to a telephone booth is provided, it should have a minimum clear width of 800 mm, although 900 mm is preferred. If doors are provided, they must not impinge upon the clear floor space within the booth (appropriately designed outward opening doors are preferred).

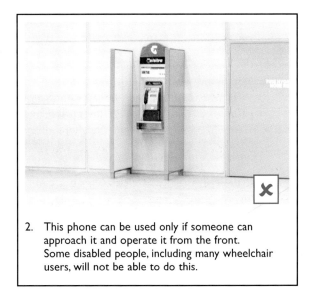

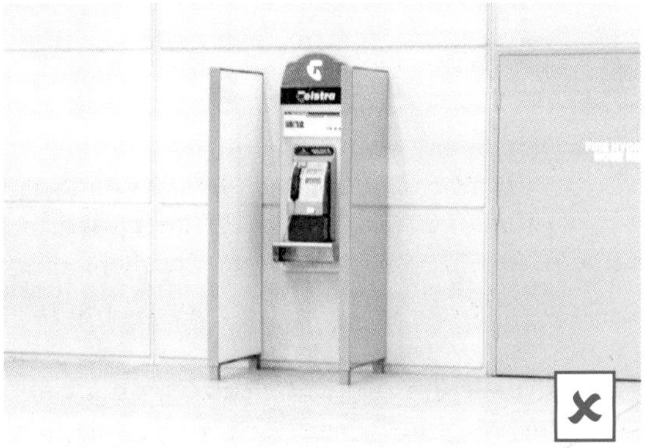

2. This phone can be used only if someone can approach it and operate it from the front. Some disabled people, including many wheelchair users, will not be able to do this.

- grab rails and shelves should be provided to give ambulant disabled people support when using the telephone

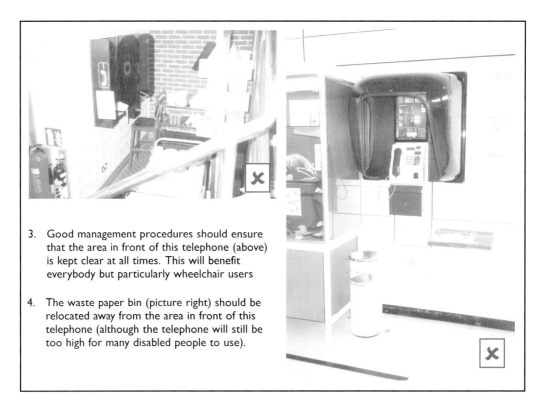

3. Good management procedures should ensure that the area in front of this telephone (above) is kept clear at all times. This will benefit everybody but particularly wheelchair users

4. The waste paper bin (picture right) should be relocated away from the area in front of this telephone (although the telephone will still be too high for many disabled people to use).

- a fold down seat (450 mm to 520 mm affl), or a perch seat (650 mm to 800 mm affl), should be provided to assist people who may find standing for a long period difficult
- telephones should be provided, or made available, for people with a hearing impairment. Such phones should be clearly marked. All public telephones should be fitted with an induction coupler which incorporates a variable volume control
- consideration should be given to the provision of text telephones (telephones which have a small visual display unit to receive messages and a keyboard to send them), at reception desks, to assist people with hearing impairments
- provision should be made for a shelf adjacent to, or associated with, all public telephones, for use by people with a hearing impairment who may use a portable text phone
- keypads should be well lit and numerals should be large and use embossed or raised figures
- instructions for using the telephone should be provided in large print format using a san serif font on non-reflective paper.

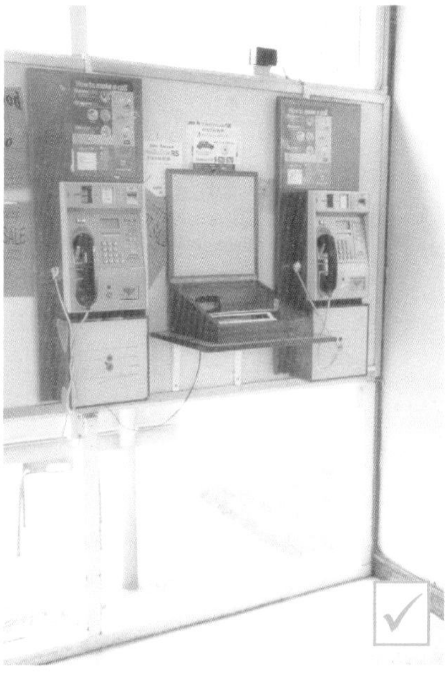

5. A text telephone will assist people with hearing problems.

14.3.3 Privacy

Acoustic hoods, if provided, must be designed and fixed so that they do not present a hazard to users. They should not project into the circulation space or, if this is unavoidable, must be suitably identified with a hazard warning.

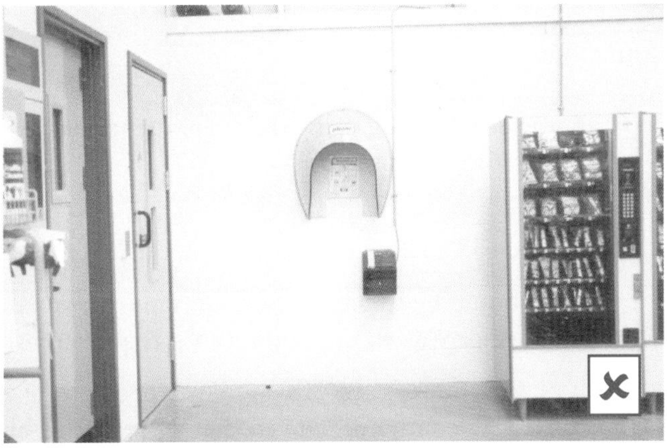

6. The telephone has been lowered but the acoustic hood has been left in the original position. This telephone is also very close to the door.

14.3.4 Telephone controls

Controls on telephones which are accessible to wheelchair users, should be positioned so that they can be used by people either standing or seated.

Controls should be located between 750 mm and 1000 mm affl and should have:

- large raised numerals
- embossed numerals
- numerals which are appropriately contrasted in terms of colour and luminance with their background
- a raised "dot" on the number 5
- well lit keypads.

14.3.5 Telephones for staff

Staff workstations should be fitted with a telephone that meets the needs of the individual disabled member of staff. Hands-free phones are particularly useful in some cases, but may not be suitable in quiet areas or where privacy is required.

There should be a text phone available for incoming calls from people who are deaf or hard of hearing, and a level of staff training to ensure there is a competent person there to use it, if required.

See 5.6.3, 14.2.2, 14.3.1, 14.3.2, 14.8.2

14.4 Water

14.4.1 Safe temperature and ease of operation

Water supplies must be delivered at safe temperatures and fittings must be easy to use and control. Disabled people with reduced sensitivity in the hands and feet are particularly vulnerable to scalding from water that is delivered to sinks, baths, basins and showers. They may also be unable to withdraw from contact with hot water, for example if bath water is found to be too hot. Water temperatures should be controlled using thermostatic mixing valves, and shower temperatures must have preset maximum temperatures.

People with restricted dexterity or arm movement will have difficulty using taps that require a twisting action to turn them on or off. Lever taps, which may also require some sideways movement but do not need a twisting action, or proximity taps, which operate when movement is detected, should be used. Clear instructions in appropriate formats are essential.

14.4.2 Water provision and delivery

In all situations:

- hot water must be delivered from the tap at temperatures that will not scald people with reduced sensitivity
- the hot water delivered from a tap operated independently by a disabled person must not exceed 41°C at the outlet
- taps should be single lever mixer taps or proximity activated taps. If individual lever taps are provided, they should not require more than a quarter turn to full flow.
- if power showers are provided, the pressure of the delivered water should be controllable and not delivered at a pressure which could cause injury or discomfort to a disabled user
- showers should be provided with clear instructions on how to use them. Control settings and symbols should be embossed and appropriately colour contrasted to assist people with restricted vision.
- a self-locating plug and chain, or a pop up waste mechanism operated with a mixer tap, is good practice, but it must be usable by people with restricted hand dexterity.

14.4.3 Improvements to existing taps

Any taps and showers that are fitted for use by disabled people must be adapted to meet their needs. Wherever possible, this should be undertaken using new purpose-designed fittings, but if this is not possible, adaptations such as extension levers to assist in turning the taps on and off, could be considered. In all cases, attention must be given to controlling the maximum delivery temperature of the water.

14.4.4 Drinking water

Drinking water, if provided in a building, must be available to all users. Drinking dispensers that use cups (preferably disposable plastic or similar), can be used by people who are unable to lean over to use a drinking fountain.

If assistance dogs accompany, or might accompany, a person into the building, facilities for gaining convenient access to drinking water for the dog must be provided.

14.4.5 Individual water heaters

Individual water heaters with maximum temperature control may be installed at the point of delivery. These installations can be energy and cost saving because they do not deliver hot water from a central source. Their design, positioning and operation, must be suitable for safe and effective use by all users, including disabled people.

See 14.2.1, 16.4.1

14.5 Gas

Users should not have to stretch to relight a pilot light, or lean over lighted cooker rings to reach other facilities, for example, a window opener.

The use of matches to light gas appliances can be hazardous for some disabled people and this must be avoided. Electronic ignition lighters should be provided wherever possible.

A person without a sense of smell may be unaware that a gas leak is occurring or that an open flue appliance is not working properly. Gas detectors and carbon monoxide detectors, with both visual and audible warning signals, should always be provided and regularly checked.

Appliances must be designed so that they cannot be misused by children.

14.6 Ventilation and air quality

14.6.1 Controllable ventilation

Ventilation into a space should be controllable and should ensure good air quality. Poor air quality and pollution can have a seriously adverse effect on some disabled people. Appropriate control is essential. This can be done either by natural or mechanical means but for the latter, the elimination of background noise is important, as is the need to ensure that fans and controls do not affect the functioning of hearing aids.

Wherever possible, ventilation in different rooms and at different workstations, should be controlled separately and, preferably, adjustable by an individual.

14.6.2 Air pollution

People who experience respiratory problems or allergies can be seriously affected by dust, tobacco smoke, chlorine and exhaust fumes. Fresh air is needed to replenish used air and to dilute pollutants. Where air conditioning or mechanical ventilation is installed, the outdoor air supply rates should be at least the level recommended in:

BS 5925: 1991 for natural ventilation

BS 5720: 1979 for mechanical ventilation and air conditioning.

14.6.3 Cleaning

Cleaning can have a major impact on air quality and can be used to improve an environment by:

- regular cleaning and vacuuming of carpets and soft furnishings
- replacing and cleaning filters in mechanical ventilation and air conditioning systems
- restricting smoking in an environment, or increasing ventilation where smoking is permitted
- ensuring windows and window furniture are properly maintained.

14.6.4 Ventilation controls

Controls for ventilation should be reachable from a wheelchair and should not require users to climb, for example onto a chair, to reach them. The use of pull cords (with bangles to assist grip), infrared hand held remote controls, or remote manually or remotely operated devices to open and close fans and windows, should always be made available where appropriate.

14.7 Heating

14.7.1 Safety and comfort

Heating equipment should be safe for individuals to operate and should provide comfortable conditions. Heating equipment should:

- not be positioned so that it causes a tripping or collision hazard

- take into account that some people, and especially disabled and older people, have sensitive skin or may have reduced sensitivity
- not have surfaces that are hot enough to burn people who touch it or stand close to it
- be provided with protecting rails or covers, if contact with a hot surface is likely
- be provided with individual controls in individual rooms and at individual workstations, reachable and suitable for all users
- not have corners or edges that could cause injury
- be recessed wherever possible and not project into the circulation space.

14.7.2 Surface temperatures

To avoid the risk of burns, the surface temperature of accessible radiators should not exceed 43°C, though this may be too high in some circumstances and may need to be adjusted to address the needs of a particular user.

14.8 Power

14.8.1 Safety and convenience

Power supplies and equipment should be safe and convenient for people to use. In general:

- while switches and sockets must be reachable by everyone, they must not be placed where children can misuse them, or where connecting cables may cause tripping hazards
- switches and controls should be easy to operate and indicate clearly positions for "on" and "off", or "high", "medium" or "low"
- equipment such as fans, compressors, computers and printers, should not produce significant background noise
- cables and equipment that create strong magnetic fields should be sited where they will not interfere with the operation of hearing aids.

14.8.2 Positions

Electrical sockets, telephone points and TV sockets, should be located at a minimum height of 400 mm and not more than 1000 mm affl. Sockets with plugs that are likely to be removed and replaced frequently should be located at the top of this range.

Switches for permanently wired appliances (such as reset switches for alarms and fused spurs), should be mounted between 750 mm and 1200 mm affl.

Light switches should be aligned horizontally with door handles to assist their location when a room is entered.

The maximum height of simple push button controls that require limited dexterity, such as isolator switches and circuit breakers, should be 1200 mm.

To assist reading, meters should be positioned between 1200 mm and 1400 mm affl. Pre-pay meters should be accessible but positioned at a height to avoid tampering by children.

Where sockets in an existing building are inaccessible and the load is small, fused and switched extension leads may be used, but trailing cables must be avoided. If necessary, sockets should be changed to types that are easy to operate. Switches on the outside of the plugs rather than between the two plugs are preferable on double sockets.

15 Evacuation

15.1 Design principles

Means of escape for disabled people comprise structural provision (for example, lifts, refuge areas, ramps), and management procedures (for example, assisted escape).

See 12.2.3

15.1.1 Safeguarding disabled people

Egress from existing buildings or environments must be considered to be as important as access into them. Both the physical features of a building and the management practices adopted must ensure that all users can egress from an environment safely and with the minimum amount of stress. Wherever possible, the aim should be independent egress.

Measures must be taken to safeguard all people using a building or environment in an emergency, whatever the reason for that emergency. This includes both disabled people (as covered by the DDA 1995), and non-disabled people who may be experiencing a more temporary need for assistance, such as people with short term injuries and women in the later stages of pregnancy. All these users may make use of a lift to gain access to the upper floors of a building, but, in most cases, will not have that particular option available to them when leaving in an emergency.

Disabled people may take longer to evacuate a building and, in many cases, will need additional assistance. This may be due to their impairment, but in some cases it will be the result of poor design of evacuation routes and inappropriate management.

In any escape strategy, it is important to offer a choice of options, and this is equally true for disabled people. The strategy should be designed to allow a flexible response to different situations without undue reliance on management procedures. However, management is the key to the effective escape for disabled people in an emergency.

It is essential that designers, building owners and mangers consider:

- how the building is being, or will be, used
- the needs of the people using the building
- the management practices and procedures that are available for implementation.

Details of structural fire protection measures incorporated in the building and proposed management practices must be made available to the users. Ensuring that disabled people are aware of the procedures that exist for emergency evacuation will greatly enhance their confidence in using the building.

15.1.2 Strategy for existing buildings

Whenever improvements or alterations are made to a building or environment, the means of escape strategies for disabled people must be reviewed. The Building Control Body should be consulted at an early stage to ensure that the work incorporates acceptable evacuation arrangements. Further guidance can be found in *Building Regulations & Fire Safety – Procedural Guidance* published by the Office of the Deputy Prime Minister (OPDM).

The code of practice for means of escape for disabled people, BS 5588 Part 8: 1988 *Fire Precautions in the Design, Construction and Use of Buildings*, acknowledges that, in existing buildings, it may not be possible to comply fully with the Code. However, it makes the important point that:

> **"non-compliance with all the recommendations of the code should not be used as grounds for excluding disabled people".**

Building managers are obliged to have a safety policy in place that considers how disabled people can be evacuated, rather than how they can be prevented from entering the building if evacuation is identified as a possible problem.

In existing buildings, it may be that the inability to achieve all the physical conditions for safe evacuation may have to be balanced with more rigorous management procedures supported by the use of better detection and warning systems.

15.2 Horizontal evacuation

The principles of horizontal evacuation are identical for both disabled and non-disabled people. Occupants of a building should be able to turn away from, or get past, danger and reach a nearby stair or exit, or a more remote stair along a protected corridor.

For disabled people unable to use the stairs, a "refuge" (see 15.4), can be provided within the same fire protected area.

15.2.1 Safe and easy routes

Generally, there should be:

- an easy and safe route on the same level within a building to a refuge or exit. Disabled people must not be expected to climb through windows, walk across undulating roofs, or negotiate steps in an emergency.
- a refuge area with direct access to an escape stair or an evacuation lift
- clear instructions and direction signs at key points informing disabled people where they should go and what they should do in an emergency
- exits designed with appropriate width, operating mechanisms, manoeuvring space and level thresholds, suitable for use by disabled people without the need for lifting or other assistance
- a "fail-safe" system that automatically releases any electronically operated locks or controls (keypads, swipe cards or proximity detectors), when the fire alarm is activated.

15.2.2 Travel distances

Disabled people can take much longer to reach safety than non-disabled people. Allowance should be made for this extra time by reducing travel distances for disabled people – especially if there is only one direction of escape. BS 5588 suggests halving the travel distance that would be appropriate for non-disabled people. In Approved Document B of the Building Regulations, a reduction in travel distance is recommended for places of assembly and recreation buildings that are primarily intended for disabled people.

15.2.3 Width of escape routes

The width of an escape route is usually determined from the guidance given in Approved Document B. Ideally, routes should be 1200 mm wide to allow for the movement of wheelchair users and other disabled people. Widths may be reduced to 900 mm, if frequent passing places of at least 1800 mm in width are provided.

15.3 Vertical evacuation

The principle of vertical evacuation is that people who are able to, can walk down (or up) through the building to a final exit where they can reach a place of safety outside the building. People who cannot negotiate stairs independently should be able to wait in a place of safety (a refuge) until they can be assisted down (or up) to the exit level. This assistance may involve the use of an evacuation lift, assistance in the use of an evacuation chair or by being carried.

Evacuation of disabled people from a basement needs to be carefully considered. It is more difficult to lift a wheelchair up stairs than to assist a downward escape. In these situations, wider stairs to facilitate lifting may be necessary.

Stair lifts and platform lifts are not suitable for evacuation. Where there are any changes in level on escape routes, there will need to be a refuge and a management procedure to facilitate evacuation.

Changes of level on fire escape routes, even if only a single step or threshold, must be avoided wherever possible.

15.3.1 Safe means of evacuation

Escape stairs, refuges, evacuation lifts and management procedures, should provide a safe means of evacuating disabled people in an emergency. Generally there should be:

- escape stairs and continuous handrails designed to meet the needs of ambulant disabled people and people with sensory impairments
- safe refuges for disabled people who cannot use the stairs
- an evacuation lift, if appropriate
- management procedures which ensure that people using refuges are assisted to safety in a manner appropriate to their needs.

See 15.6.3

15.4 The "refuge concept"

The British Standard Code of Practice for means of escape (BS 5588 Part 8: 1988), emphasises the role of management practices in escape arrangements for disabled people. The code gives guidance on means of escape in all premises other than dwellings, and introduces the concept of refuges and the use of an evacuation lift.

Refuges are areas within a building that have been designed and designated as protected spaces where disabled people can wait to be assisted to the final exit from the building. They should be positioned so that a disabled person can access them without changing floor levels. Routes to refuges should be short enough to be negotiated quickly, or they should be protected from fire. Except for very short routes, there should always be alternatives.

Generally, refuges should meet the following requirements:

- be in an escape staircase or have direct access to one
- have enough space for one or more wheelchair users to wait without encroaching on the escape route. It is often the case that one refuge per stair is provided at each floor level. However, there may be situations where larger refuge areas would be required, for example, where the number of disabled people using the building is high.
- be clearly signed and identifiable
- have clear, easily legible instructions in appropriate formats
- have an appropriate means of two-way communication
- have space for storing assistance equipment, such as Evac chairs, if required.

All refuges should be fitted with a two-way communication system suitable for use by any disabled person. A CCTV system is also strongly recommended. The provision of both will not only assist the disabled person in what will be a traumatic experience, but will also help fire and rescue services to identify that refuges are occupied and attend to those first.

If there is insufficient space in an existing building for a refuge within the protected stair enclosure, extending the protected enclosure, perhaps by repositioning a fire door or moving partitions, may be possible. Borrowing space from an adjoining room, building a platform over a stair well, or rearranging the escape route where a stair may be wider than necessary, are options for ways of creating space for a refuge in an existing building.

See 12.2.3, 15.2.1, 15.3,15.6.3

15.5 Assisted escape

Some form of assisted escape is likely to be needed from most public access buildings and from buildings where disabled people are employed. It is important that disabled people are consulted and contribute towards the development of suitable evacuation plans for an individual building or environment. However, the needs of visitors will not always be known and strategies must be developed to accommodate their evacuation needs.

When designing an evacuation plan, it is important for the disabled person to be asked about their abilities, and to avoid making any assumptions. For example, a disabled person may not need to be carried simply because they are a wheelchair user. Some wheelchair users can walk short distances, or may have other ways of effecting their escape that they are quite happy with.

When an evacuation plan is developed, there will often be a need to appoint assistants or to request volunteers, sometimes called "buddies", to help in emergencies. This presents a much better management policy than looking for assistance only when it is needed.

Situations that need careful consideration may arise when the disabled person:

- does not have one particular workplace
- wishes to work out of normal hours.

Some disabled people could be seriously injured if they were lifted, and this is particularly relevant for some wheelchair users if they are lifted from their chairs. Management strategies for escape must never allow for the lifting of a wheelchair or any disabled person, unless the staff carrying out the lifting have been appropriately trained. Wheelchair users must be consulted before being lifted.

Any proposal for lifting within an evacuation strategy must take into account relevant health and safety legislation, such as that related to lifting regulations in the workplace.

15.6 Evacuation techniques

15.6.1 Phased evacuation

The term "phased evacuation" is used when the people in an area most immediately affected by a fire (usually only the floor affected by the fire and the one above), are evacuated first, together with any disabled people in the building. This principle would be used principally in large existing buildings, hospitals etc, but could be adopted for most building types.

15.6.2 Zoned evacuation

This technique is used generally in large buildings where evacuation from the affected area is by moving people horizontally into adjoining fire protected areas. This type of evacuation might be used in shopping centres because it reduces the need for assistance for disabled people as they can still use any lifts in the unaffected areas.

15.6.3 Evacuation by evacuation lift

In some buildings, it is essential that evacuation lifts, purposely designed to include a role in emergency evacuation, are provided. The lift requires a "protected lobby" with direct access to a stairway, and should be operated only by management in the event of an emergency. The lobby area could be used as a refuge area and, ideally, should be fitted with a two-way communication system and CCTV.

Evacuation lifts, as described in BS 5588 Part 8: 1988, are usually passenger lifts that have their own separate or back-up power supply. When evacuating a building, a designated and appropriately trained member of staff should facilitate escape using the passenger lift. The Fire and Rescue Service may assist in this if appropriate. A lift may be suitable for use in an evacuation if:

- it has a direct exit to a place of safety at the final exit level
- it has a lobby on the upper or lower floors separating the lift entrance door from the rest of the floor
- the lobby has a space for a disabled person to wait without obstructing the escape route
- both the lift and the lobby are contained within fire resisting construction, unless the lift or lobby forms part of a protected shaft, in which case a higher fire resistance may be required
- the lobby doors have an appropriate fire rating
- the lift has an independent power supply that will not be interrupted if the power in the building is switched off
- the lift has a switch at the exit that overrides the landing call buttons and puts the lift under the control of the floor level selector buttons in the car
- there is a communication system in the car that can be activated from each lobby to inform the car operator about which floor a disabled person needs to be evacuated from.

The standards of provision and the limitations on the use of a lift for evacuation purposes must be agreed with the fire officer for each particular building.

Even where an evacuation lift is available for use by disabled people, there should be an escape stair, with refuge, also provided for use if the lift fails.

15.6.4 Discarded wheelchairs

In an emergency evacuation, a wheelchair may be discarded after a disabled person has been assisted to safety. This may be particularly so in places of mass assembly, such as sports stadia or auditoria. Management policies must allow for discarded items such as wheelchairs which can block the evacuation route of other users, and ensure that staff facilitating escape are trained to identify any potential dangers and deal with them.

15.7 Provision of information

Disabled people should be provided with information that enables them to take their own actions, as far as possible, for securing escape in an emergency. Insufficient information for any user can lead to irrational or panic behaviour that can seriously affect any existing escape strategies for the building.

Asking disabled people to wait in a refuge area while everyone else escapes will undoubtedly cause them stress. This can be reduced if there are management procedures in place and disabled people are kept fully informed of events. They will be reassured if they know that:

- others are aware of their presence and position in the building
- others are aware of their particular needs with regard to assisted escape
- two-way communication is available within the refuge
- the scale of the fire does not threaten them
- fire-resisting construction separates the refuge from the fire
- procedures have been regularly practised and everyone is aware of what is required.

15.8 Fire engineering approach

Fire engineering is based on:

- assessing the risk of fire breaking out in any part of the building
- predicting the size and type of fire that would develop
- defining strategies that would reduce the effect of the fire on occupants and property.

It differs from a prescriptive fire safety approach in that it is not based on a set of rules, but rather on balancing active and passive protective measures to reduce risks to an acceptable level.

A fire engineering approach can provide the basis for designing protected escape routes and for Personal Emergency Egress Plans (PEEPs). Fire safety engineering can take into account things that reduce risk such as:

- staff training
- detection and alarm systems
- pressurisation to prevent spread of smoke
- good internal communication systems.

If a fire engineering approach is proposed, it is essential that it is discussed with building control or an approved inspector at an early stage.

15.9 Personal Emergency Egress Plans (PEEPs)

These should be developed as part of a management procedure after full consultation and agreement with the disabled people who will be using the building. PEEPs are used mainly where the needs of an individual are known, such as in an employment situation. A PEEP should be provided for all disabled people who have an impairment for which some assistance will be required to evacuate the building in an emergency.

The plan should take into account:

- the type of building
- the design of the building
- what difficulties may be encountered when escaping in an emergency
- the type of assistance needed to overcome those difficulties
- any other requirements specific to that person or employee.

In public access buildings where the individual evacuation needs of people using the building may be more difficult to determine, a variation of a PEEP, known as a Standard Evacuation Plan should be developed.

15.10 Routes of escape

It is important to provide people with the information they need so they can understand the routes they need to take to escape from the building. In some existing buildings, or if evacuation lifts are provided, disabled and non-disabled people may need to travel in different directions. Routes must be provided with clear, unambiguous signs.

Instructions must be provided in appropriate formats (size of text, font, reflectivity of surface etc), so that they can be used by disabled users who may wish to escape using the main escape routes.

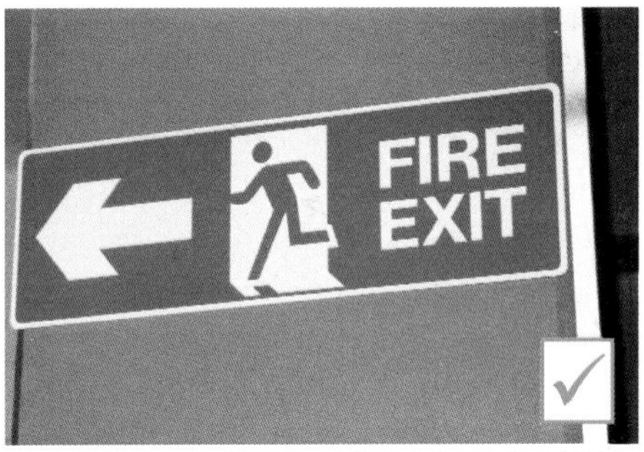

1. To avoid confusion, information should be clear and appropriately placed.

See 3.8, 3.9, 15.1, 15.1.1, 15.1.2, 15.2.1, 15.2.2, 15.2.3, 15.5, 15.7

15.11 Automatic control of fire doors

Fire doors, which can be heavy and difficult to negotiate, can present a barrier to accessibility because, for them to function properly, they need to be closed when a fire occurs. Any fire door that has to be manually opened to proceed along a route can present particular problems for disabled people. However, movement around a building can be enhanced for many disabled people if fire doors are held open on electromagnetic catches linked to the fire alarm system. Hold-open devices must be linked to an alarm incorporating Automatic Fire Detection (AFD), typically smoke detectors. Many fire alarm systems do not incorporate AFD. When the alarm is raised, the catches are released and a door closer shuts the door. It is important that the release mechanism operates on a fail-safe system, so that if the power supply fails, the door automatically closes.

When carrying out an access audit of a building it is important to check that disabled people can open the doors if they return to the closed position. If not, people may become trapped within an area that they were previously able to enter with ease.

An electrically powered hold-open device, conforming to BS EN 1155, should be installed on doors where the closing force at the leading edge of a door on a circulation route exceeds 20 Newtons.

If electromagnetic hold-open devices are not used, it is important that adjustable powered door closers are provided. These closers will allow adjustments to be made to meet the minimum door closing force recommended in BS 8300: 2001, and ensure the correct operation of the door. Some power units may provide a closing force which is different from that recommended in BS EN 1154, which requires a minimum closing force of 18 Newton metres. The use of cam action door closers can offer greater flexibility in addressing this problem.

15.12 Alarms

The code of practice for fire alarm systems is BS 5839: Part 1 2002, with some elements covered by BS EN 54. Fire alarm systems consist of:

- detectors and call points that alert management to the outbreak of a fire
- warning or communication systems that alert occupants when there is a need to evacuate all, or parts, of the building.

Both of these factors can cause difficulties that need to be addressed when ensuring appropriate emergency egress from an existing building for disabled people.

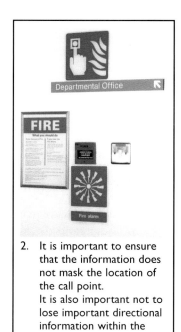

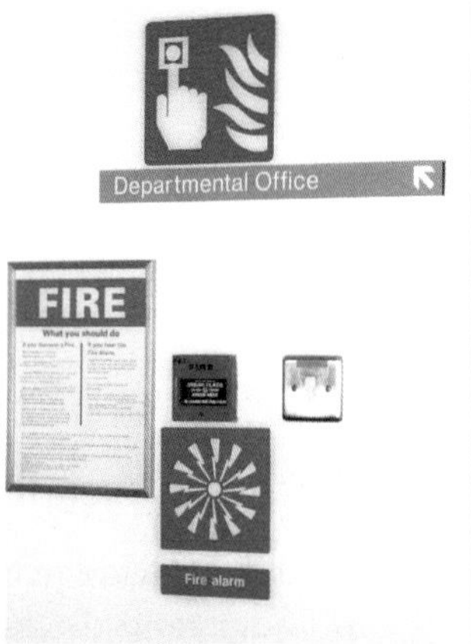

2. It is important to ensure that the information does not mask the location of the call point.
It is also important not to lose important directional information within the more "visually obvious" fire information, or to place important features, such as light switches, too close to call points.

15.12.1 Communication

Warnings and instructions must be clear and unambiguous, provided early in the escape process and in appropriate formats. Flashing lights or illuminated signs that are activated at the same time as any bells or public address systems, should be provided to alert people who are deaf or hearing impaired.

The current British Standard for Fire Safety Signs Notices and Graphic Symbols (BS 5499 Part 1: 1990), does not address signs specifically intended for the evacuation of disabled people. Some fire officers accept a combination of standard fire safety signs with the international access symbol. Procedures for evacuation need to be clearly displayed in alternative formats at key points.

15.12.2 Raising the alarm

The fire alarm system in a building should be suitable for everyone. Generally:

- manual call points should be located where all users can reach them. If appropriate, consideration should be given to providing alternative types such as pull cords.
- call points are usually 1400 mm affl and often require the breaking of a glass panel which can be difficult for some disabled people
- the recommended travel distance to a call point of 30 m will need to be reduced if it is expected that the alarm could be activated only by a person who has restricted mobility

- any two-way communication systems located near call points, must be suitable for people with sensory impairments
- alarms should always be visual and audible in all parts of the building
- fire fighting equipment should be positioned to allow easy operation by everyone
- fire alarm systems should be used only in a fire and during planned testing of the equipment.

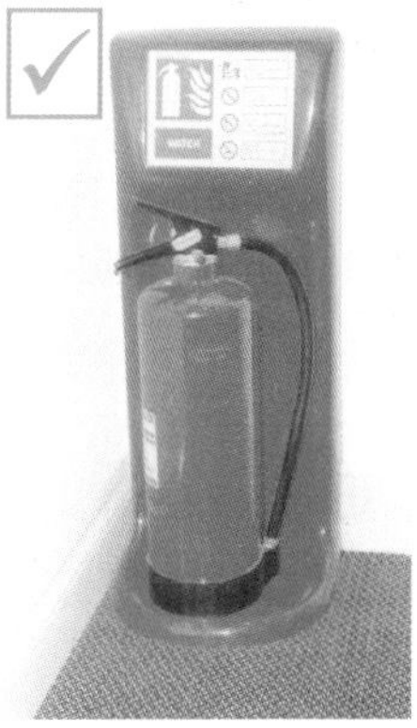

3. An example of fire equipment that is easy to use by most people. It does not project into the corridor and cause an obstruction.

The following examples represent the type of equipment that can assist management in developing an evacuation plan. These can also be used to support the provision of PEEPs:

Sound alerter

– this works in conjunction with a fire alarm system to send out directional sound frequencies to assist the listener in identifying the route to follow.

Security systems

– these include modern security systems, such as those requiring security card entrance into certain parts of a building or environment that can be used to locate people if an emergency occurs

Evac chair

– a folding chair with sledge type runners that some wheelchair or ambulant disabled users can transfer into and be transported downstairs to an exit point. They are not suitable for all wheelchair users, such as those with neck and spine injuries.

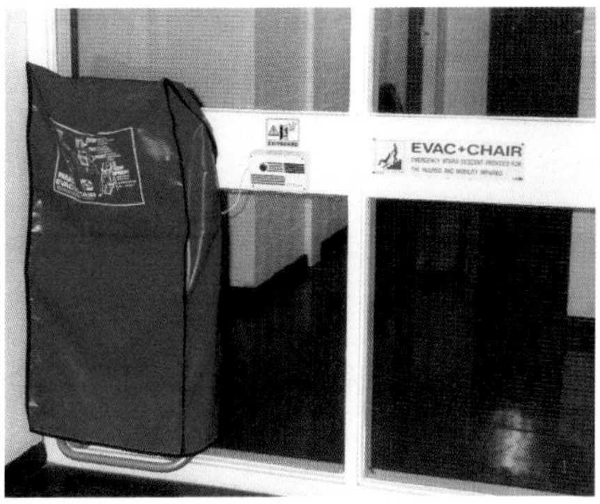

4. The use of an Evac chair can assist some wheelchair and ambulant disabled people when evacuating a building. It is important that management procedures are in place to ensure that staff know how to use the Evac Chair.

Flashing beacons

– these should be provided in all areas where a person is likely to be alone and/or where they will not hear the fire alarm, perhaps if they are deaf or hard of hearing

E-alert

– these are modern systems which can be used to alert people by flashing a light or message when activated by the alarm system. This can be particularly helpful to people who are deaf or hard of hearing.

Telephone systems

– these can be used to alert people by flashing lights or ringing

Vibrating pagers

– these are used to alert people who are deaf or hard of hearing when the alarm has been activated. Maintenance, retrieval and how they are used, all need careful consideration.

CCTV

– if part of a security system, this can be used to monitor areas such as refuges

Powered and unpowered wayguidance systems

– these may assist the efficiency of evacuation in a large area, for example auditoria, theatres and cinemas.

15.12.3 Public address systems

Automatic public address systems or "voice evacuation systems" are linked to the fire detection system and offer an alarm system which is less reliant on staff intervention. These systems can assist disabled people by giving different instructions to those with different needs, perhaps directing some people to refuges and others to the stairs.

It is important that all audible information is supported by visual information.

See 15.12.1

15.13 Emergency and escape route lighting

There are several regulations and standards concerned with the provision of emergency lighting in buildings. The Building Regulations 1991, Approved Document B, details fire safety requirements for new buildings and has been revised and issued as Edition 2000. This identifies the locations that must be provided with emergency lighting, although special premises such as sports grounds and sub-surface railway stations have their own regulations.

In general:

- all open areas other than residential sites larger than 60m^2, must be provided with emergency lighting
- emergency lighting is now needed for all parts of schools that either do not have natural light or are used outside normal school hours.

The Fire Precautions Act 1971, modified and extended by the Workplace Regulations 1997, covers all areas where people are employed, except for special premises.

Generally:

- where five or more people are employed, a formal record of Fire Risk Assessment must be kept. Compliance with BS 5266 (EN1838) (BSI, 1999a) is deemed to comply with these requirements
- the illuminance requirements in BS 5266 Pt 7 (EN1838) 1999 calls for a minimum of 1 lux anywhere on the centre line of the escape route for normal risks.

The UK has an "A deviation" to continue to allow a 0.2 lux minimum in routes that will be permanently unobstructed. In this case, the user must ensure routes are kept clear at all times, even in an emergency. For this reason ICEL recommends that the 1 lux level should always be used.

15.13.1 Specific design guidance for accessibility

Emergency lighting must be designed to operate automatically when required. The design and installation of emergency lighting systems is controlled by a highly prescriptive set of standards and regulations. To provide an accessible environment, the design should be compliant with the regulations and standards, and take into account the particular needs of people with low vision.

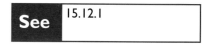

15.13.2 Overhead emergency lighting

For people with limited vision, overhead emergency lighting systems should provide 3 lux along the centre line of the escape route (floors and stairs) (Webber *et al*, 1997). This is greater than the minimum illuminance recommendation of 0.2 lux in British Standard BS 5266. For overhead emergency lighting:

- emergency lighting luminaires should be positioned out of people's direct line of sight to reduce glare (particularly at the bottom of stairs)
- uniform lighting should be provided to reduce adaptation problems
- the escape route through a space lit by overhead emergency lighting is provided by exit signs. Internally illuminated exit signs assist in identifying the route.
- internal surfaces of the space should be provided with adequate contrast, particularly on stairs, at doorways and at changes of direction
- the escape route must not be visually cluttered or obstructed.

15.13.3 Powered wayfinding provision

These systems are included in BS 5266 and offer an alternative means of providing emergency lighting and wayguidance along an emergency escape route. In general, they are produced in a strip or track that can be placed along the escape route at either floor or skirting board level.

Systems can be non-powered (for example, photoluminescent material) or powered (for example, light emitting diodes).

Emergency lighting systems and signs that use only photoluminescent material are inadequate for people with low vision.

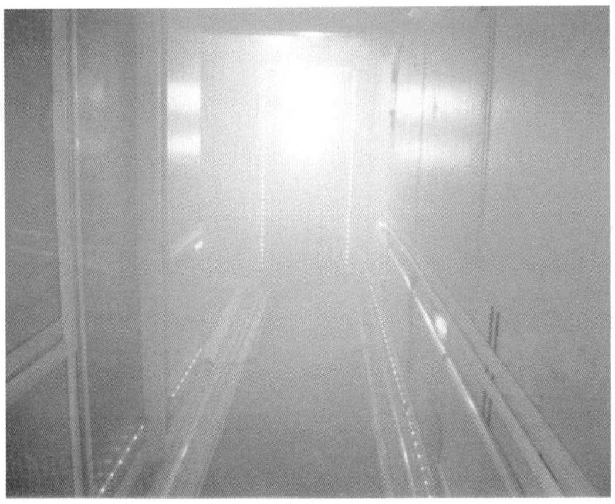

5. Light emitting diodes in a smoke filled corridor.

15.13.4 Design overview

In general:

- people with visual impairments have a preference for systems that combine wayfinding systems with basic overhead emergency lighting
- the minimum illuminance on the floor for combination systems should be the same as for wayfinding systems: at least 0.3 lux on the centre line of level parts of a route and at least 1 lux on a stair
- apply the ICEL guidance, particularly the requirement for 1 lux on the centre line of an escape route
- total reliance on a photoluminescent material to define an escape route should be avoided
- adequate contrast of the building fabric particularly at stair nosings, doorways and changes of direction is essential
- when using emergency lighting, people with visual impairments prefer to have handrails on both sides of a stair, irrespective of the width.

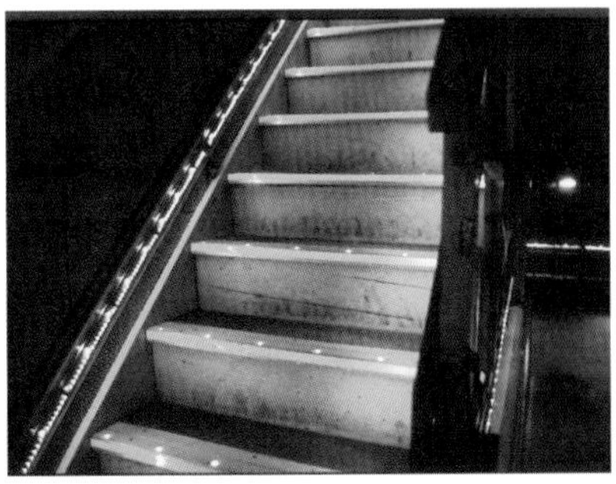

6. Light emitting diodes highlighting the route and the nosings of the treads.

See 13.11

16 Facilities

16.1 Design principles

16.1.1 Availability, standard and use

All facilities should be accessible for independent use by disabled people. A disabled person attending an event such as a theatre or sports meeting as part of a group, should be able to sit with his or her companions.

Wherever possible, facilities for disabled and non-disabled people should be sited together and the provision should always take into account that the gender of a disabled person's carer may not be the same as that of the disabled person. This is particularly important with regard to changing rooms or toilets.

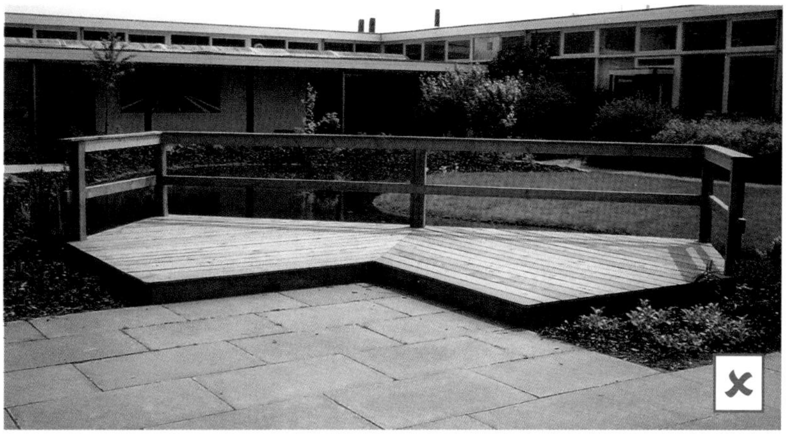

1. Equality of access should be considered in the provision of all facilities. Here a viewing and leisure platform has been constructed, but it is not accessible to disabled people.

16.2 Accessibility

16.2.1 Public accessibility

In many situations, there are tangible benefits to building owners, managers, service providers and employers, in making their buildings and environments as accessible as possible. More customers, opportunities to hold a wider range of events, fewer home visits, increased flexibility in the use of premises, good publicity generated by an inclusive approach and access to a wider talent in the workforce, are all potential benefits.

The accessibility of any one facility has to be considered in the context of the building or environment as a whole. All users attending the theatre, for example, or a restaurant, bar or transport facility, would expect to find toilet provision. They would also expect to use other associated facilities such as ticket offices and promotional shops in the theatre or cafeterias, and shops in transport environments. In a leisure centre, all users would expect to be able to access showers, lockers, swimming pools, sports facilities, gyms, spectator seating, solariums and vending machines. Disabled people are no different in this expectation, nor should they be.

If provided, all facilities must meet the needs of all potential users. While, in existing buildings, some compromises may be necessary, using the inability to implement full accessibility as an excuse for doing nothing is never acceptable.

16.2.2 Accessibility for employees

The DDA protects disabled people from discrimination in the field of employment (both opportunities and prospects for progression), and as part of this protection employers may have to make "reasonable adjustments" if their employment arrangements or premises place disabled people at a substantial disadvantage compared with non-disabled people. Where necessary, premises should be adapted to ensure this is possible.

In exceptional circumstances, where access to a building – or part of a building – cannot reasonably be achieved, employers are expected to review their management practices, policies and procedures to see if alterations can be made to overcome any physical barriers. This could include, for example, offering a different working place, perhaps in another building.

In terms of employment, it may not be necessary to make all parts of a building or environment fully accessible if access to them is not an integral part of a disabled person's employment duties. However, working towards full accessibility of an environment should always be the aim.

What must be emphasised is that the employment opportunity, while not necessarily identical, must be equal in all respects.

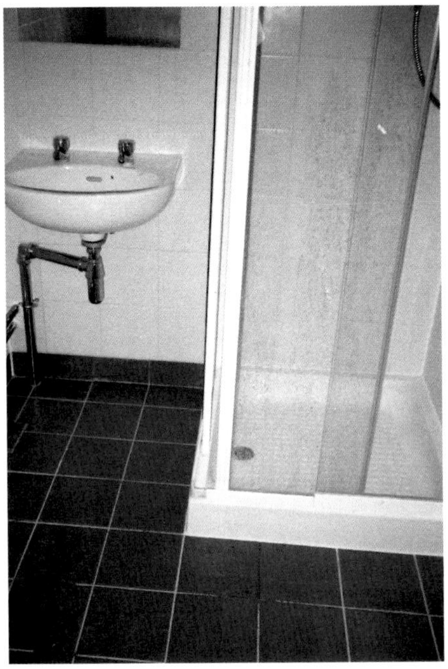

2. A shower facility has been provided for staff, but it is not accessible for all existing or potential employees because of the upstand.

The wash basin height and the use of twist style taps may also affect use by some disabled people.

If a disabled person who could not use this facility was employed, this would not be seen as an equal provision.

See 4.1, 4.1.3, 4.3.1, 4.3.2, 4.4, 4.5, 4.7.4, 4.7.6, 8.2.1, 12.2.3, 13.1.1, 15.13.1

16.2.3 Routes to toilets

Routes giving access to toilet facilities must always be kept clear of obstructions, be as direct as possible and of an appropriate width (see Chapter 11).

In an employment situation, the travel distance to an accessible facility should be decided in accordance with the individual needs of the disabled employee. However, in no circumstances should that distance exceed:

- 100 m on the same floor level
- a total of 40 m of horizontal travel if the journey includes both horizontal and vertical travel (by accessible lift).

A disabled person should not have to travel more than one storey to reach a suitable toilet.

Floor finishes, such as deep pile carpets, can have a considerable detrimental effect on the ability of a disabled person to move around a building. This must always be taken into account when deciding appropriate travel distances.

16.3 General toilet facilities

For many building users, the accessibility of an environment will be determined by their ability to locate and use toilet facilities. Wherever possible accessible toilets should be sited close to other toilet facilities and not be tucked away nor look like an afterthought.

Whilst accessible toilets are designed to meet the needs of wheelchair users, many other people (rightly or wrongly), also use them. The additional space is particularly useful for people with assistance dogs, older people, people with luggage, or parents with pushchairs. Unfortunately, this demand reduces the availability of the accessible toilet for wheelchair users. Managers of environments must ensure this does not happen. Designers should allow for larger cubicles in standard toilet accommodation because they address the needs of many users.

See 6.3.6, 16.1.1, 16.2.3, 16.3.1, 16.3.3, 16.3.5, 16.3.7, 16.3.8

16.3.1 General guidance for toilet facilities

Generally:

- doors and lobbies should be designed to allow easy access to all WCs
- sanitary fittings should be colour contrasted with the background against which they will be viewed
- fittings such as door locks, dispensers and flushes, should be usable by people with restricted mobility and dexterity
- surfaces should be slip-resistant and non-reflective
- cubicles should be large enough for comfortable use, especially if the door is inward opening
- one or more larger cubicles should be provided for situations when more space would be desirable, such as for use by parents with children, users with assistance dogs, people with luggage etc
- lighting should be 100 lux minimum (see also Chapter 13).

Modesty panels between urinals can assist men with visual impairments to orientate themselves and, if provided in addition to colour contrast, can considerably improve accessibility.

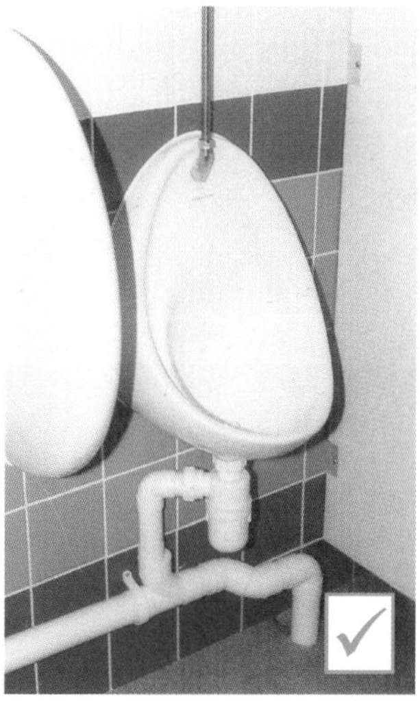

3. Good colour contrast can improve accessibility considerably, and at no additional cost. Modesty panels are also useful in assisting men with a visual impairment to orientate themselves correctly at the urinal.

The time taken to travel to any toilet is a critical consideration when deciding where it is located in an existing building.

If there is only one accessible toilet suitable for wheelchairs and ambulant disabled people in a building, this should be a unisex facility.

In existing buildings, where there may be restricted space at entrance level or on any level that is accessible to wheelchair users, separate gender standard toilet accommodation should contain at least one larger cubicle with accessible facilities.

There is no published standard for the number of accessible toilet facilities to be provided in a building. The appropriate number should relate to the type and use of the building. However, at least one accessible unisex toilet facility should be provided at each location in a public access building where toilet provision is made available for the use of customers and visitors.

The provision of accessories available within an accessible toilet facility, for example, shaving points, vending machines etc, should be:

- the same as that provided in other standard toilet accommodation, or
- provided in an area which is accessible to both disabled and non-disabled people (perhaps a lobby area).

Disabled people should have access to facilities that are of an equal standard, especially in terms of standard of finishes, convenience and usability.

16.3.2 Toilets for ambulant disabled people

A minimum of one cubicle designed to meet the needs of ambulant disabled people should be provided in each male and female toilet facility.

Generally, the toilet should have:

- internal dimensions of at least 1500 mm by 800 mm
- a cubicle door that opens outwards. Where an inward opening door is unavoidable, the length of the cubicle should be increased to ensure that there is at least 450 mm clear space between the door swing and any internal fitting
- horizontal grab rails (as shown in Figure 16a)
- at least one urinal fitted with vertical grab rails each side.

Lobbies and doors giving access to the toilets containing cubicles and urinals for ambulant disabled people should be designed to ensure easy access.

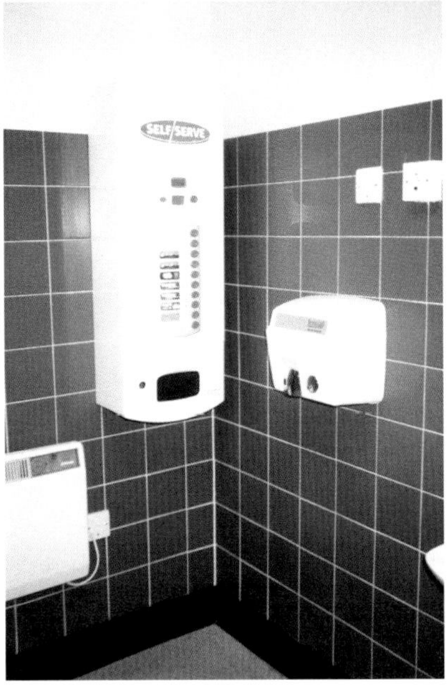

4. If vending machines are available for use by non-disabled people, they must be equally available for use by disabled people.

   Disabled people do shave, some use feminine hygiene products and some use condoms. They would like the same opportunity to buy them as anyone else.

16.3.3 Wheelchair accessible toilet

An accessible toilet should be provided in conjunction with an accessible route. Toilet facilities suitable for use by ambulant disabled people should always be provided in standard toilet facilities, even if they are not accessible to wheelchair users.

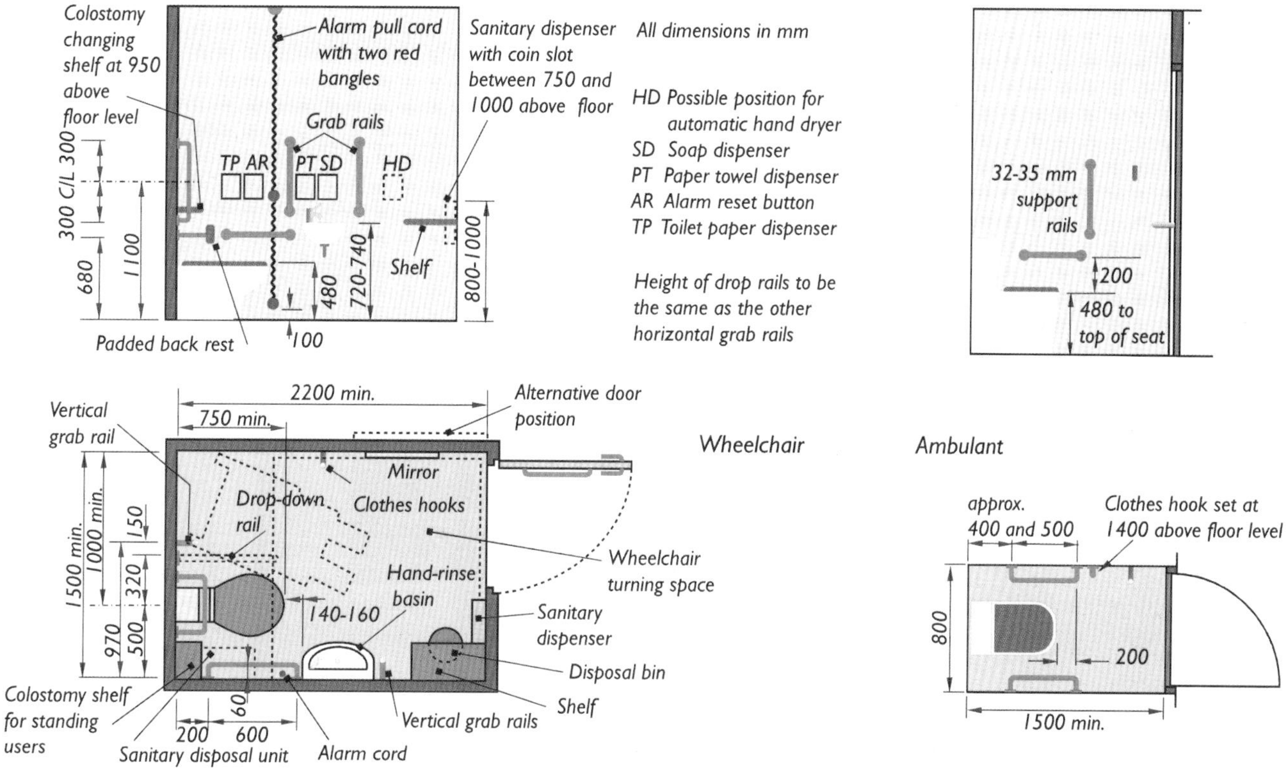

Figure 16a Recommended toilets for wheelchair users and ambulant disabled people.

Generally:

- if only one accessible toilet is provided it should be unisex. This will allow a carer of the opposite gender to the disabled person, to go into the accessible toilet without having to go through standard male or female toilet accommodation.
- the distance that a disabled person should be required to travel from their work position to the nearest accessible toilet should be decided relevant to their individual needs (see 16.2.3)
- the provision and location of accessible toilet facilities should ensure that both disabled people and non-disabled people are equally well served
- doors and lobbies should be designed to allow easy access to all WCs.

There should be sufficient space to allow people to transfer onto the toilet. People may transfer from the left or right hand side, or the front of the WC. The direction of transfer may be determined by a particular impairment, the pain caused as a result of transferring, or because some people feel safer and more confident transferring in a particular way.

BS 8300: 2001 states that: "Right hand transfer is taken to mean transfer to the right when a person is seated in their wheelchair".

Where only one wheelchair accessible toilet is provided, service providers must be aware that some disabled people may be unable to use the facility. Where two or more wheelchair accessible toilets are provided, a choice of left and right hand transfer should always be available. In an employment situation, accessible toilet facilities should be provided only once the needs of particular employees are known by the employer (see 16.3.7).

Service providers and employers must consider whether the level and appropriateness of the provision available could be viewed as reasonable under the obligations imposed by the DDA in each individual circumstance.

The layout of wheelchair accessible toilets, and the placing of fixtures and fittings, should conform with the recommendations of BS 8300: 2001, shown in Figures 16a.

Generally wheelchair accessible toilets should have:

Visibility

- wall and floor surfaces which are non reflective
- sanitary and other fittings which contrast in terms of colour and luminance with their background.

Ease of approach

- easy to open door furniture
- appropriate width to the approach corridor or lobby.

Usability

- minimum internal dimensions of 2200 mm by 1500 mm. These minimum dimensions must not be compromised by wall finishings, skirting boards etc
- fittings such as soap dispensers, toilet paper and paper towels should be suitable for single-handed use and for use by people with weak arm movements. These fittings, together with the washbasin, must be positioned so that a disabled person can use them safely whilst seated on the WC.
- toilet paper should be provided in a single sheet dispenser. Large toilet paper dispensers and those with serrated edges for tearing paper must be avoided
- drop down rails must be easy to operate and fitted so that they do not need lifting before being lowered

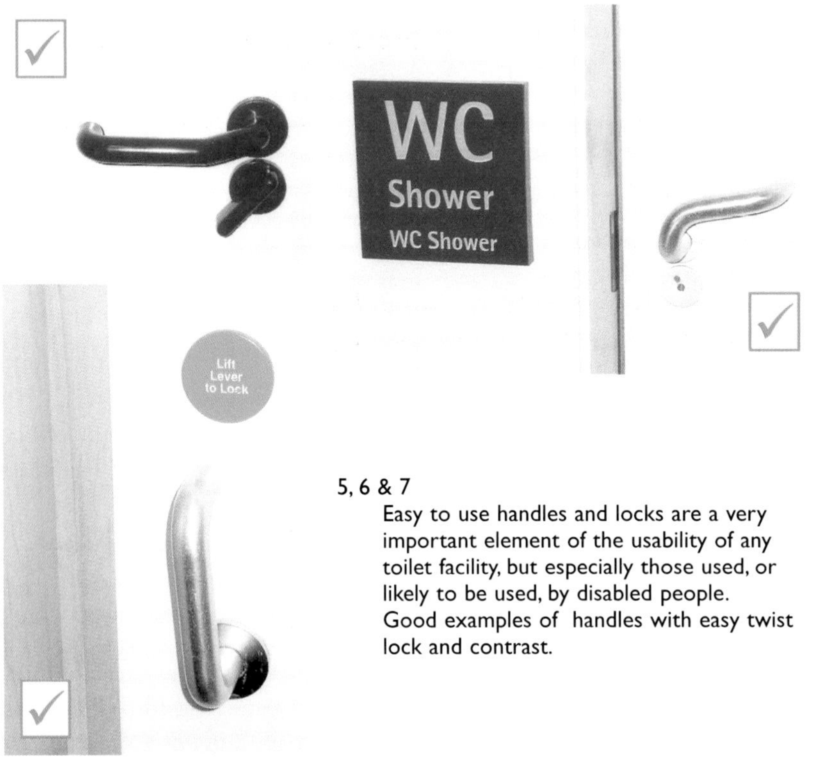

5, 6 & 7
Easy to use handles and locks are a very important element of the usability of any toilet facility, but especially those used, or likely to be used, by disabled people. Good examples of handles with easy twist lock and contrast.

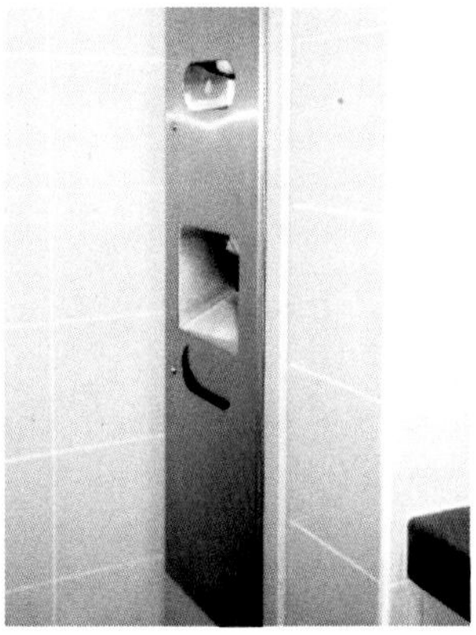

8. All facilities should be accessible, including all elements of hand washing or hand drying equipment.

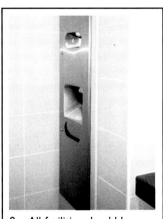

- a lever type flush with a spatula style handle should be provided and always located on the transfer (open) side of the cistern
- sealed containers for disposing of incontinence pads and other disposable items should be provided. They must not encroach into the manoeuvring space.
- coat hooks should be provided at 1050 mm and 1400 mm affl
- a mirror should be provided above the washbasin, fixed close to the top of the basin, and extend to 1600 mm affl

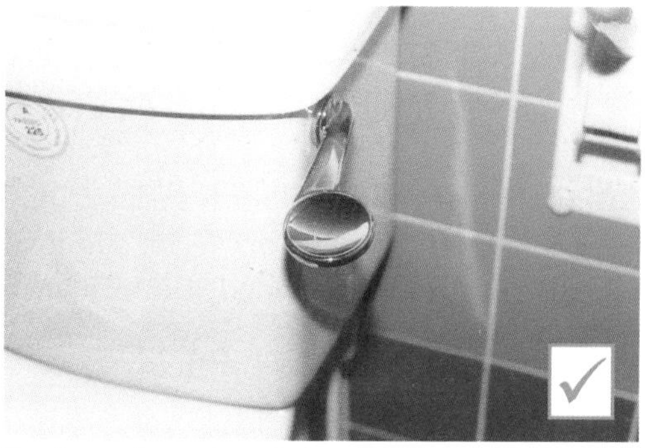

9. A good spatula style handle. This handle can be used with a closed hand, arm or elbow.

- if a mirror is positioned away from the washbasin, it should be at least 1000 mm high and set with its bottom edge at 600 mm affl
- a shaver point should be provided adjacent to the mirror and between 800 mm and 1000 mm affl
- a shelf, 400 mm wide and 200 mm deep, set 700 mm affl, should be provided adjacent to the washbasin. Care should be taken to ensure that the shelf does not encroach into the manoeuvring space.

Good communication

- projecting signage to identify location of the toilet
- visual and audible alarm indicators.

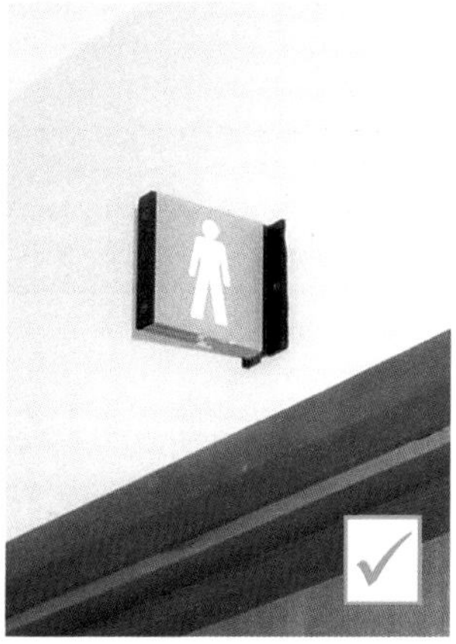

10. Good use of projected signage and symbols.

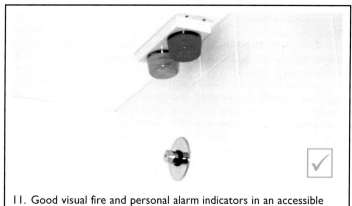

11. Good visual fire and personal alarm indicators in an accessible WC.

Safety of use

- an outward opening door allows access to the toilet if a disabled person falls against the door. If the door must open inwards, the internal manoeuvring space must be a minimum of 700 mm by 1100 mm, and the door must be fitted with hinges or fittings that allow access from the outside in an emergency.
- heated driers, if provided, which are operated by a push button, rather than proximity movement detectors
- floor surfaces should be slip resistant

- seats with a gap at the front should not be used
- taps should be either single lever mixer taps or proximity taps which deliver water at a controlled temperature (not exceeding 41°C at the outlet).

"Peninsular" toilets, which allow transfer from both sides and supported by drop down rails, are not suitable for use in public access or employment situations and must be used only where skilled assistance is also provided. Peninsular toilets must never be provided as a substitute for two separate, unisex WCs.

An accessible toilet should be fitted with a means of calling assistance in an emergency. A pull cord, red in colour, and capable of being operated from the WC or the floor, should be provided. The cord should have two "bangles" (50 mm diameter), one set at between 800 mm and 1000 mm affl, and the other set at 100 mm affl.

If the alarm is activated, both audible and visual indication should be given inside the toilet. This is particularly useful if the alarm has been accidentally activated. A reset button, which can be reached when seated on the WC or in a wheelchair, should also be provided.

The alarm should:

- be connected to a staffed security or reception desk
- activate a visual and audible alarm outside the toilet (in a position that will be seen or heard by others)
- have an audible sound that is unique and easily distinguishable from any other alarm sound.

Management procedures must be put in place to identify the course of events when the alarm is activated, and who is responsible.

Accessible toilets must never be used as storage areas, even if the area is larger than required.

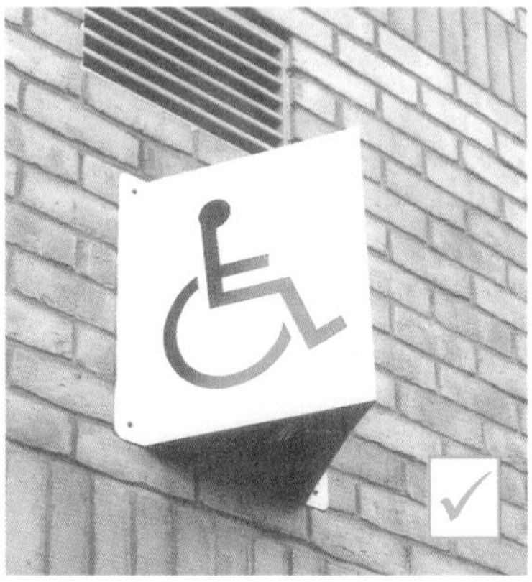

12. A good protruding sign to allow the location of the accessible toilet to be identified from a distance.

16.3.4 Baby-changing facilities

Baby-changing facilities should not be located in an accessible toilet where there is only one accessible compartment. If provided, baby-changing facilities should be accessible to both male and female carers and be usable by both disabled and non-disabled people.

Fold down baby-changing benches are often left in the down position. This can seriously encroach into manoeuvring space and management procedures should be introduced to address this issue.

16.3.5 Toilet facilities for working assistance dogs

If people with assistance dogs are employed or use a service within an existing building, an external area of 2000 mm by 3000 mm minimum should be designated for use by working dogs.

The facility should include:

- a sign indicating that the area is designated "For assistance dogs only"
- a suitable surface of grass or bark chippings

- a supply of plastic bags and a dispenser
- a hand washing facility, if possible
- a management procedure for cleaning and maintaining the area.

16.3.6 Public access toilets

If only one accessible toilet is provided:

- there is no published guidance on whether the facility should provide for a left or a right hand transfer. In such circumstances, it may be necessary to be guided by the ease of installation and ensure that there are no projections into the manoeuvring space by, for example, pipes.
- publicising the direction of transfer of the accessible toilet on promotional literature or a web site, if available, will allow disabled people to decide whether the toilet facility is one that they can use and enable them to plan their visit more carefully.

16.3.7 Accessible toilet facilities in the workplace

If only one accessible toilet can be provided, installing a facility without knowing the needs of the employee might result in expensive rework. In such situations, it would be better to identify a suitable area where the toilet could be provided, have the management procedures in place to move swiftly, and have the money available to pay for the work if required.

16.3.8 Controlling access

One of the disadvantages of publicly accessible toilet accommodation is that the larger internal space can be inappropriately used. This may include people sleeping in the facility, or using the space for drug abuse. In some public areas, controlling their use of accessible toilets may be difficult. Overhead ultra violet lighting used to deter drug abusers from injecting, can render the accessible WC virtually impossible to use for a person with a visual impairment.

Wherever accessible toilets are provided, management should consider:

- how to ensure that the toilet is available for use by disabled people when required
- where there is controlled entry, for example by locking the facility when not in use, how access to the key can be readily available when needed
- whether a RADAR KEY control be fitted.

The RADAR KEY is a national scheme operated by the Royal Association for Disability and Rehabilitation (RADAR) and its purpose is to prevent unauthorised or inappropriate use of accessible toilet facilities. Unfortunately, whilst RADAR key locks are common, not all disabled people are key holders. If this facility is provided, procedures must be put in place to ensure that disabled people can obtain a key if required. Disabled people should never be required to travel long distances to obtain a key. RADAR key locks should be unnecessary if the WC is managed and monitored appropriately, for instance, in shopping centres or community buildings.

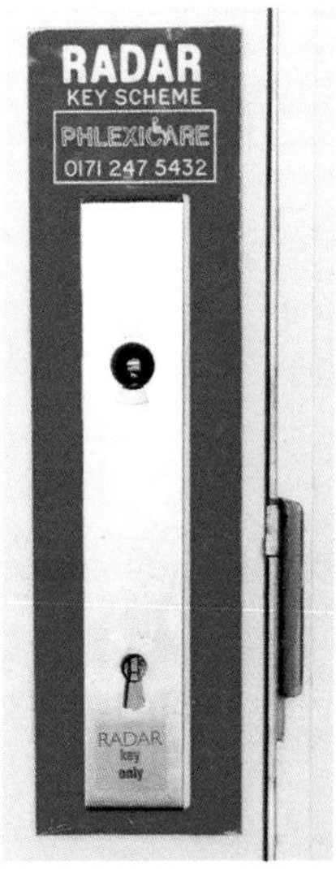

13. A RADAR key facility

16.4 Accessible showers and bathrooms for independent use

No single design or layout will meet the needs of all disabled people. However, many needs can be addressed if a variety of bathroom layouts are provided, for example with an integral WC which allows for alternative directions of transfer.

The following guidance relates to non-domestic buildings such as hotels, halls of residence and some sports buildings.

The number of shower and bathroom facilities accessible for use by disabled people should reflect the numbers of disabled people likely to require such facilities.

16.4.1 Safe and convenient use

Generally:

Visibility

- the general lighting in a bathroom should be between 100 and 300 lux
- lighting should not produce glare
- wall and floor surfaces should be non-reflective
- fittings should contrast in terms of colour and luminance with their background.

Ease of approach

- showers and bathrooms should be conveniently located close to, and on the same level as, areas used for sports facilities, changing rooms and bedrooms
- there should be sufficient manoeuvring space inside and outside showers and bathrooms, and the areas should be served by doors that are wide enough to allow independent use by wheelchair users.

Usability

- where only one accessible bedroom with an en-suite bathroom is provided, the bathroom should incorporate a shower (rather than a bath), because some disabled people are unable to use a bath
- where there is more than one accessible bedroom with en-suite facilities, there should be a choice of bath or shower and a choice of left or right hand transfer to the WC
- all accessible bathrooms and showers should contain a WC
- showers should be fitted with a tip-up seat, grab rails, and a shower curtain enclosing the seat
- a shelf should be provided for toiletries
- safe, dry, and lockable storage facilities should be provided close to the bath or shower
- taps and shower controls should be suitable for the needs of people with restricted manual dexterity, and dispense water appropriately.

Good communication

- bath and shower rooms should be fitted with a means of calling assistance in an emergency. In bathrooms it should be reachable from the bath.

Safety of use

- floors to accessible showers and bathrooms should be level and all showers and bathrooms should be provided with surfaces that are slip resistant when wet and dry
- where the shower tray forms part of the floor finish, a slight fall towards the gulley will be required
- seats should be provided and grab rails should be installed to assist people both when standing up and sitting down
- baths should have a flat slip-resistant base, a transfer seat, a rim height of 480 mm and a horizontal or angled support rail.

16.4.2 Dimensions

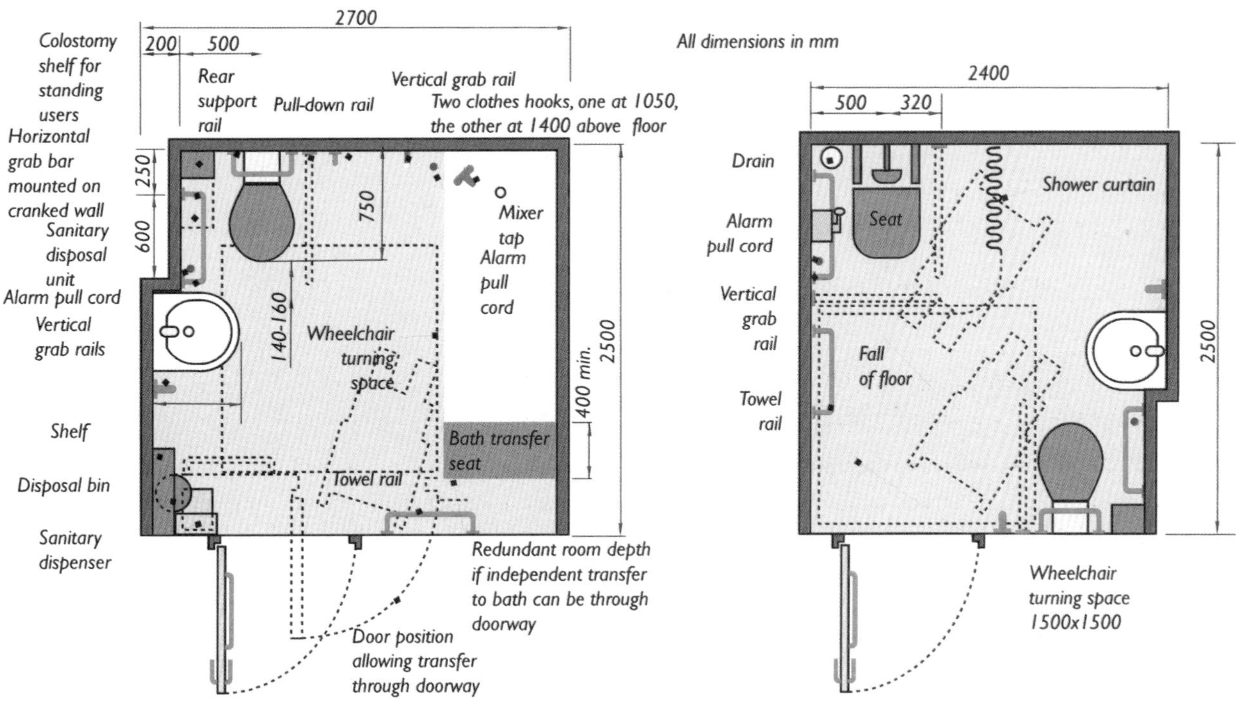

Figure 16b Shower and bathroom for wheelchair users.

The size and layout for showers and bathrooms are shown in Figure 16b. Level access throughout is essential. Detailed guidance is given in BS 8300: 2001.

16.4.3 Hospitals and residential homes

Specific requirements for showers and bathrooms, where there is assisted use, are contained in BS 8300: 2001.

16.5 Accessible changing rooms

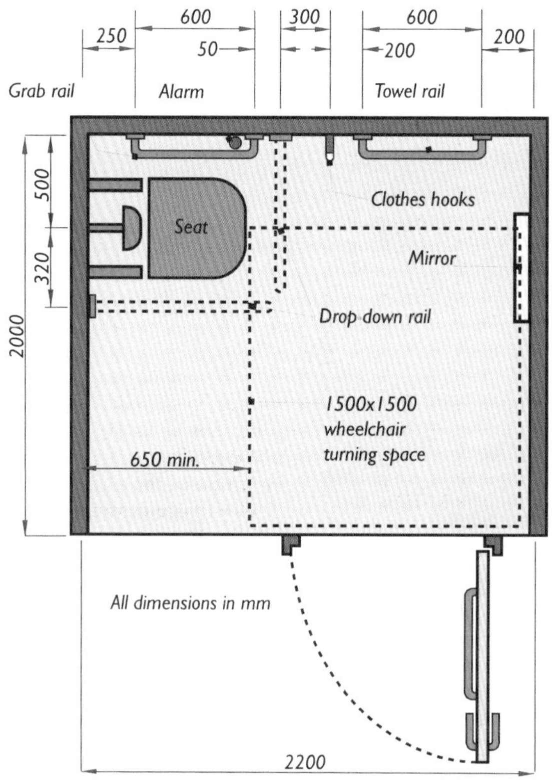

Figure 16c Self-contained changing area and accessories.

The needs of disabled people using changing facilities will vary but, in most cases, they can be addressed with good, flexible, management practices, and an appropriately trained staff.

16.5.1 Safe and convenient use

Changing rooms should:

Visibility

- have non-reflective surface finishes
- be appropriately lit without glare
- have good colour and luminance contrast of fittings with their background and at the floor/wall junction

Ease of approach

- be conveniently located for related activities and have corridors and doors that are wide enough for disabled people to use. In some cases, corridors and doorways will need to be wider to take into account the additional width of sports wheelchairs.
- be provided with locks and latches that are easy to operate and can be opened from the outside.

Usability

- ensure privacy of changing with cubicles large enough for wheelchair users, curtains and wide doors
- be accessible to both genders (so that an assistant of one gender can help a disabled person of the other)
- be provided with lockers that are reachable and have some lockers that are large enough to store artificial limbs or callipers.

Good communication

- have visual and audible alarm indicators.

Safety in use

- have floor finishes which are slip-resistant when both wet and dry.

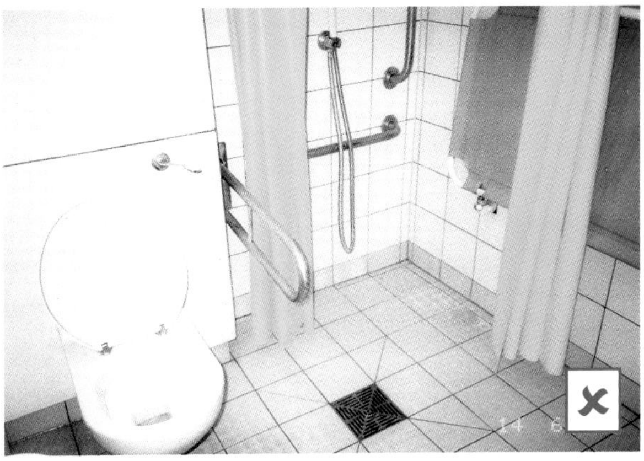

14. A combined toilet and shower facility (above). The position of the gulley in the centre of the floor may mean that a large area of the floor remains wet, and potentially hazardous. There is also no shelf for toiletries and a drop down seat has not been provided.

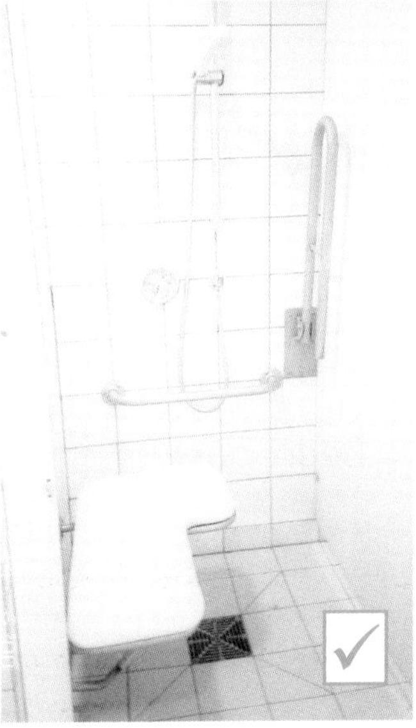

15. A shower (right) with a drop down seat provision.

16.5.2 Lockers

All lockers should be appropriately constructed and situated in dry areas adjacent to the changing rooms. There should always be sufficient unobstructed manoeuvring space (minimum 1500 mm by 1500 mm), between and in front of lockers.

Lockers:

- provided for wheelchair users should be a minimum 300 mm wide by maximum 600 mm deep, and with the base of the locker between 400 mm and 800 mm affl
- intended to store crutches, callipers or artificial limbs should be a minimum of 1200 mm high
- intended for walking frames should be 800 mm by 600 mm in plan area
- should have locks that can be easily operated by one hand and be no higher than 1150 mm affl.

The provision of large lockers is important. In an existing facility, it may not be necessary to change all the lockers provided that some larger ones are available, and disabled people have priority in their use.

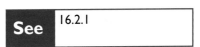

See 16.2.1

16.6 Cloakrooms

This section covers only the facilities available for visitors to leave and collect property that they do not wish to take into an existing building.

16.6.1 Convenient and useable

Generally cloakrooms:

- should be conveniently located, with level access and adequate manoeuvring space for all users
- self-service fittings and storage equipment should be reachable
- secure spaces should be provided to accommodate temporary storage of large personal items, such as wheelchairs and walking frames, if required.

16.6.2 Provision

All cloakroom fittings must be designed to meet the needs of disabled people and the amount of accommodation provided must reflect the expected, or potential demand. Management procedures to ensure that assistance is available for disabled people, if required, must be seen as additional enhancement that is available to all users, not as a substitute for poor provision.

16.7 Provision of wheelchairs

In some buildings, for example museums, exhibition buildings, hospitals and shopping centres, wheelchairs may be made available to people who find travelling over longer distances difficult. A designated space should be provided which will allow wheelchairs to be stored away conveniently, without encroaching into circulation space.

16.8 Bedrooms

This section includes only bedrooms for hotels, motels, hostels, residential and nursing homes, university and college halls of residence. It does not cover specialised bedroom design, or bedrooms in private houses, which must be designed when the individual needs of the disabled user, are known.

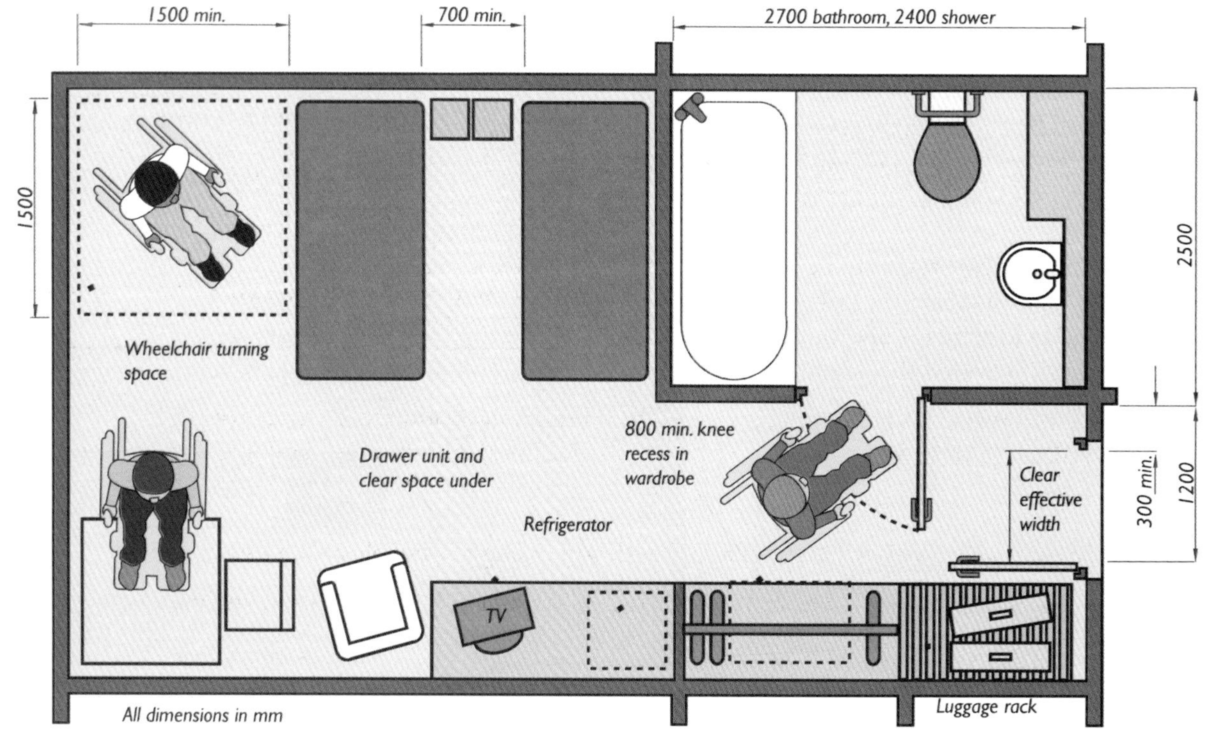

Figure 16d Example of twin bed accessible bedroom.

Full accessibility, with appropriate manoeuvring space, need be provided only in designated accessible bedrooms. However, wheelchair users should be able to enter any bedroom as a visitor to the occupants of the room. Some disabled people will need to bring assistance dogs with them into bedrooms.

An accessible bedroom should cater for as wide a range of needs as possible.

The numbers of accessible bedrooms should reflect the number of disabled people likely to use the facility, and other activities occurring within the building. However, a minimum of one accessible bedroom should be provided for every 20 standard bedrooms, or part thereof.

Wherever possible, an accessible bedroom should have a connecting door to an adjacent bedroom, for use by the companion or carer of the disabled person.

16.8.1 Strategy in existing buildings

Where space is limited in an existing building, it may be possible to improve accessibility, particularly in double rooms, where table and chairs can be moved to increase manoeuvring space. Positioning beds against a wall may increase usable floor space, but there may be difficulties in making the bed.

16.8.2 Accessible and useable

Bedrooms should be accessible, designed and managed to allow independent use wherever possible. Some bedrooms must be suitable for use by disabled people. This will include sufficient manoeuvring space, appropriate use of colour and luminance contrast, good lighting provision and the provision of usable, accessible fixtures and fittings.

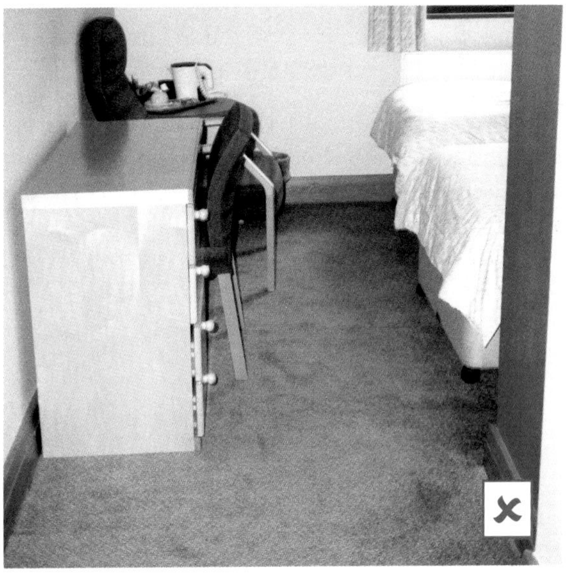

16. There is insufficient space in this room for manoeuvring a wheelchair. However, this is available as an accessible bedroom.

In general:

Visibility

- bedrooms should be provided with good lighting and colour and luminance contrast

Ease of approach

- manoeuvring space should be sufficient to allow easy and safe transfer between the bed and a wheelchair and to use storage facilities
- accessible bedrooms should be in a convenient position in relation to other bedrooms and facilities in the building (for example, sports facilities, dining rooms and lounges).

Usability

- beds should be at a height of 480 mm affl and firm enough to enable safe transfer
- a clearance of 150 mm should be provided to accommodate the supports of a mobile hoist
- accessible bedrooms should have a dedicated (preferably en-suite) accessible bathroom facility
- accessible bedrooms should have sufficient space to allow for access and use of sitting areas, balconies and desks for writing, if provided.

Good communication

- telephone facilities, if provided, must be suitable for use by people with sensory impairment
- TV sets should be capable of receiving information in subtitles and text
- a TV listening aid should be available if requested
- an alarm system for use in emergencies should be provided with call points in both the bedroom and the bathroom facility.

Safety of use

- beds in accessible rooms should have legs positioned at each corner only, and an uninterrupted space between them (to allow the use of a mobile hoist)
- all controls for lighting, ventilation, heating, radio and TV etc, should be reachable from both the seated and the standing position
- provision should be made to ensure that lights can be reached and operated from both the seated position and from the bed
- alarm systems should be visual and audible. Vibrating alarm systems should be available on request.

16.9 Refreshment areas

16.9.1 Accessible and useable seating

Disabled people should have access to all seating areas, but not necessarily all the seating in an area. There should be a choice of seats both with and without arms, and with different seat heights. Seating should be robust enough to allow a person to use the arms for assistance when sitting or standing.

Disabled and non-disabled people should have equal access to areas that are classified as:

- self-service/waited service
- smoking/non-smoking
- outside/inside
- families with children/no children
- upper level/lower level
- with view/without view
- lights refreshments only/full meals.

Some seating should be moveable to allow space to be made for wheelchair users, or people with restricted mobility. When fixed seating is provided, suitable integrated spaces should be provided at a number of tables. Circulation routes should not be used for this purpose.

Gangways between tables and at payment points should be at least 900 mm wide to allow for unobstructed access.

16.9.2 Suitable facilities

All public facilities provided in restaurants and bars, such as telephones, toilets, vending machines and self-service counters, should be accessible to disabled people. Appropriate management procedures and staff training at self-service facilities are essential because some disabled people who use mobility aids, or people with restricted strength, may be unable to carry trays,.

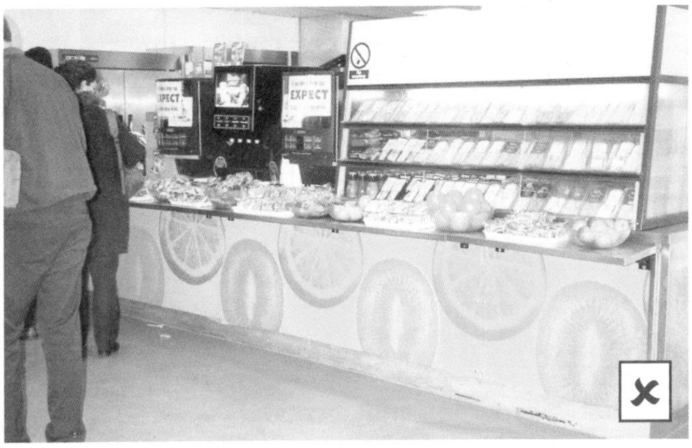

17. Disabled and non-disabled people would find this servery very difficult to use.

The tray slide has been used as an additional sales area and the vending machines are very difficult to reach, especially when holding a tray.

Till displays should be visible to assist disabled people when purchasing items. This is particularly helpful for people who are deaf or hearing impaired, as they will be able to follow the transaction and see the total price without asking questions or "hearing" answers. Interference from electrical equipment usually makes induction loops ineffective at payment points.

16.10 Retail areas

16.10.1 Accessible and useable

Generally:

- counters, vending machines, displays, gaming tables and change machines, should be accessible to disabled people
- consideration should be given to stacking items vertically on a series of shelves, rather than horizontally on one shelf. This will make items more accessible to a greater number of people.
- gangways, including checkouts in self-service and supermarkets, should be wide enough to be used by disabled people
- all gangways and checkouts should have level, slip-resistant flooring
- signage should be clearly visible when either standing or seated
- shopping trolleys should be provided that are suitable for use by wheelchair users or ambulant disabled people
- in retail stores with more than one floor, a passenger lift should be provided in addition to any stairs or escalators
- for larger shops there should be suitable parking and accessible toilets. Other facilities, if provided, such as a coffee bar, crèche or customer advice points, must be accessible to disabled people.
- staff should be appropriately trained to assist if requested.

16.10.2 Smaller retail outlets

In smaller shops, the essential features are a level entrance, a counter that has a lowered section (800 mm affl), and management policies designed to address the provision of assistance for disabled people. Aisle widths are usually critical in smaller premises. Increasing the width of the aisles may reduce selling space to such an extent that the business becomes no longer viable.

Under the DDA, commercial factors such as this could be considered as a justification for smaller retailers not to make the shop fully accessible. However, management procedures would need to be in place so that inaccessibility is minimised and, wherever possible, consideration should be given to providing the service by reasonable alternative means. Each case would have to be considered on individual circumstances – there is no "one size fits all" solution.

Where part of a shop is inaccessible to disabled people, and it would be unreasonable to rectify the situation, management policies on how to provide the most appropriate service and staff training, are critical.

16.11 Spectator areas

16.11.1 Suitable provision and access

Suitable access and provision of seating and spaces for wheelchairs and assistance dogs should be provided which allows disabled people the same opportunity to view an event as that offered to non-disabled people. People who use assistance dogs need space clear of the gangway, for the dog to lie down. Tall people, or people with restricted leg movement, will also require additional legroom.

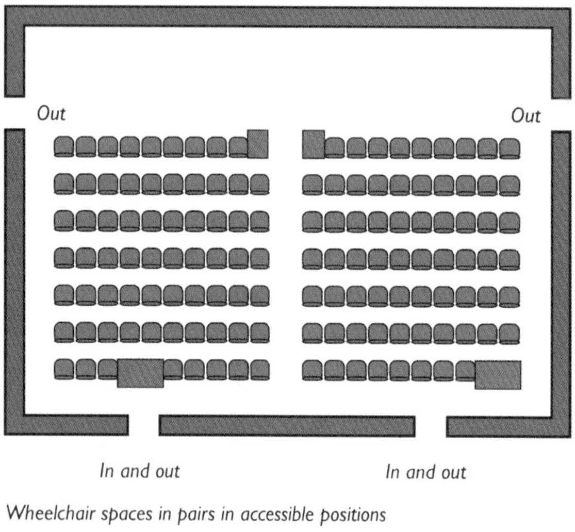

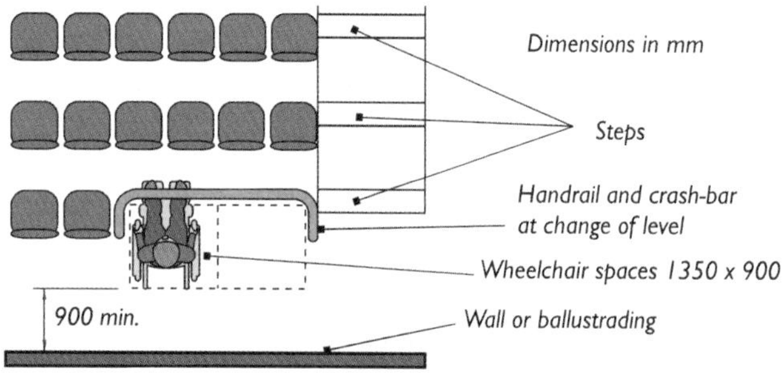

Figure 16e Distribution of wheelchair spaces in an audience.

Subtitles and sign language interpretation should be provided if required.

Generally:

- accessible spaces for disabled people should have a clear view of events and performances
- seating for disabled people should not obstruct participants or other members of the audience
- accessible seating areas should be designed so that spectators in wheelchairs can still see the event, even when located behind standing accommodation or when people in front may stand up
- sight lines should allow people to view projection screens, high level electronic text devices and sign language interpreters
- there should be a choice of seating position. Accessible spaces should not be available only on the corners of seating areas or only in the back or front row, but also integrated into different parts of the auditorium. Choice is an important issue for disabled people, as it is for non-disabled people.
- a variety of seating both with and without arms, and seat height, should be provided wherever possible
- performances and announcements should be available in alternative formats such as audio support, and supported by sound enhancement systems such as induction loops, or infrared systems
- seating for disabled people should be provided so that the disabled person can sit either with disabled, or non-disabled companions.

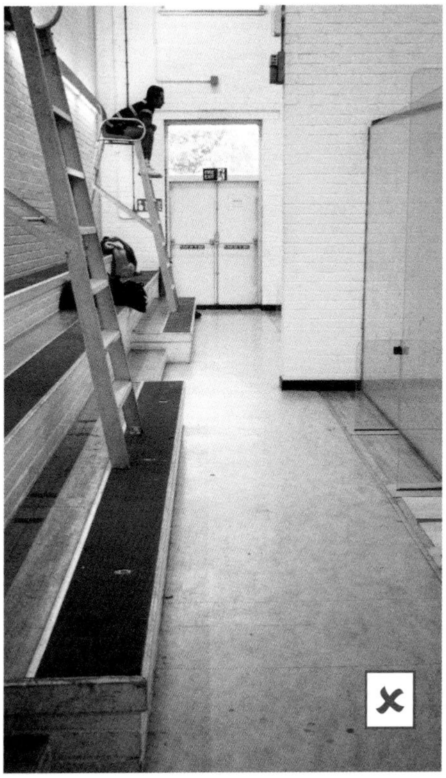

18. Spectator seating for squash courts. Where would a wheelchair user sit here without blocking the important fire escape route?

16.11.2 Strategy for existing buildings

It may not be possible to achieve the ideal choice of seating positions for disabled people. However, permanently removing some seats, or making some seating easily removable can increase the options available for different seating configurations.

In some existing buildings, it may be practicable only to provide accessible seating areas on the entrance level.

Ambulant disabled people may have difficulty getting into seats in a closely packed auditorium and getting down into the seat or rising from it, if the seat does not have arms.

Spaces or seats adjacent to gangways may have the extra space disabled people need. Consideration must also be given to ensuring that circulation routes are kept clear at all times.

It is important to ensure that accessible seating is not regarded as being isolated, or appearing just as an addition to the front, side or back of the auditorium. It is also important to ensure that, wherever possible, a disabled person can sit with either disabled, or non-disabled companions.

Sound enhancement systems and sign language interpretation can be provided in most existing buildings.

16.11.3 Management

Information about the venue and the facilities for disabled people should be made available in alternative formats. Booking arrangements should ensure that accessible seating spaces, and the spaces adjoining them, are not allocated to non-disabled people before all other seating has been allocated.

16.11.4 Further guidance

Detailed guidance relating to the provision of spectator and other seating is given in BS 8300: 2001.

16.12 Access for disabled people who are participants

Facilities should be provided at all sports venues for disabled people to participate in any sport that is available, and at all levels of competition.

Sports wheelchairs, which are generally wider than other wheelchairs, require a clear opening door width of 1000 mm for convenient access. This must be taken into account at entrances, circulation routes and in gaining access to associated facilities, such as refreshment and social areas.

Detailed guidance on the design of swimming pools, fitness suites and exercise studios for disabled people, is given in *Access for Disabled People*, published by Sport England.

16.12.1 Swimming pools

Generally:

- there should be level access between the changing facilities and the pool areas
- unisex changing facilities should be designed to allow for assisted changing
- direction and information signs should be increased in size to assist those users whose vision is reduced because they are unable to wear their glasses when using the pool.

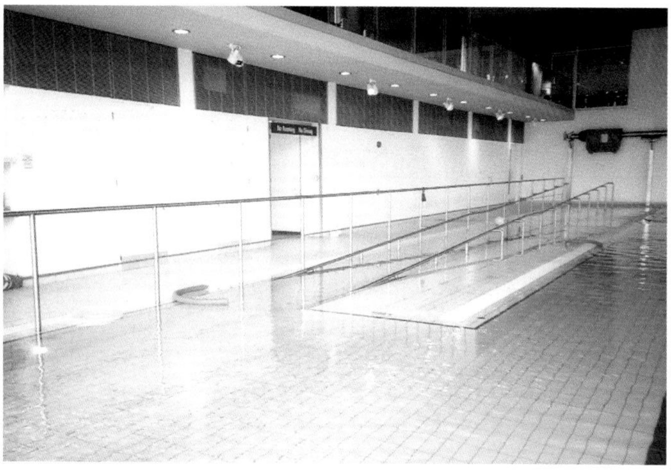

19. Good accessibility into the pool.

16.12.2 Fitness suites and exercise studios

Disabled and non-disabled people should have equal access to the same fitness and exercise areas.

Sound enhancement systems should be provided to assist people with hearing impairments to receive any music or instructions being offered.

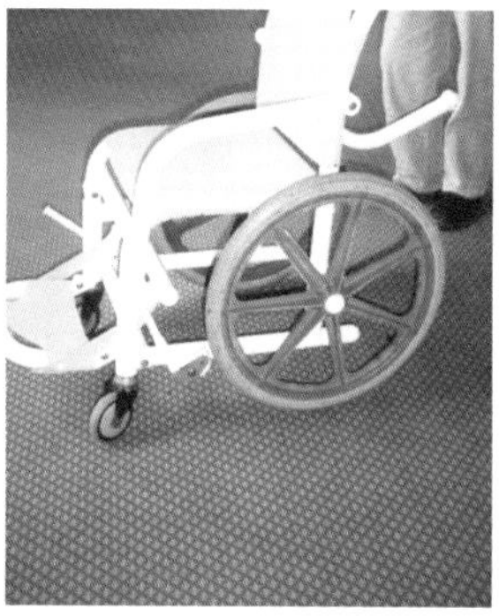

20. Leisure facilities, such as this one in Australia, may also provide wheelchairs to be used in the pool.

16.13 Meeting rooms

This section deals with rooms used for meetings or other exchanges of view, such as discussions, debates, trials and tribunals.

16.13.1 Design principles

Meeting rooms should enable full participation by disabled people.

Generally:

- all meeting rooms should be fully accessible
- the environment should enable people to communicate with others or to receive information from them
- disabled people, including wheelchair users, should be able to reach the speakers' platform, the dock, the witness box, the jury box, the public gallery, or any other part of the room available to non-disabled people
- wherever possible, any different levels within the meeting room should be accessible
- seating should have integrated positions that disabled people can use comfortably
- lighting should be well designed and address any risk of glare
- sound enhancement systems should be provided
- a selection of positions for use by a sign interpreter should be identified.

16.13.2 Strategies for existing buildings

If disabled people are unable to access all parts of an existing meeting area, arrangements must be made to ensure they can still participate as fully as possible.

If ramped seating is provided, access to only the lower or the upper section may be acceptable, but care must be taken to ensure that disabled people can comfortably see and/or hear what is happening, and be able to participate if he or she wishes to do so.

Appendices

A Information sources

Legislation, codes and standards

Copies of the following legislation are available from The Stationery Office and can be viewed on www.legislation.hmso.gov.uk

The Disability Discrimination Act 1995 (DDA)

The Disability Right Commission Act 1999 (DRCA)

Special Educational Needs and Disability Act 2001 (SENDA)

Statutory Instruments

Statutory Instruments under the DDA can be viewed at www.legislation.gov.uk

Codes of practice, standards and other associated legislation

Code of Practice, Rights of Access, Goods, Facilities, Services and Premises,
The Stationery Office (2002)

Code of Practice, Elimination of Discrimination in the Field of Employment against Disabled Persons or Persons who have a Disability
The Stationery Office (1996)

Code of Practice, Duties of Trade Organisations to their Disabled Members and Applicants
The Stationery Office (1999)

Code of Practice for Schools
The Stationery Office (2002)

Approved Document to Part M, 1999, Access and facilities for disabled people, DETR
The Stationery Office

Approved Document to Part M, 2004, Access to and use of buildings, DETR
The Stationery Office

BS 8300:2001, Design of buildings and their approaches to meet the needs of disabled people
Code of Practice, BSI, 2001

BS 5588:Part 8:1988, Fire Precautions in the design, construction and use of buildings
Code of Practice for means of escape for disabled people, BSI, 1988

Human Rights Act, 1998
The Stationery Office

Equal Treatment Directive, 1975 (Amended 2002)
The Stationery Office.

B Useful organisations and contacts (in alphabetical order)

Organisation	Contact
The Access Association	01922 652 010 www.accessassociation.co.uk
Building Cost Information Service Ltd (BCIS)	Tel: 020 7695 1500 www.bcis.co.uk
British Standards Institution (BSI)	Tel: 020 8996 9000 www.bsi-global.com
Cadw: Welsh Historic Monuments	Tel: 029 2050 0200 www.cadw.wales.gov.uk
Centre for Accessible Environments	Tel and minicom: 020 7357 8182 www.cae.org.uk
Chartered Institute of Building Services Engineers (CIBSE)	Tel: 020 8675 5211 www.cibse.org
College of Occupational Therapists	Tel: 020 7357 6480 www.cot.co.uk
Department for Transport, Mobility and Inclusion Unit	Tel: 020 7944 3000 www.mobility-unit.dft.gov.uk
Disabled Living Foundation	Tel: 0845 130 9177 www.dlf.org.uk
Disabled Persons Transport Advisory Committee (DPTAC) This site hosts the DPTAC Access Directory. The Directory has been set up to offer free advice on published guidance in the area of accessibility and inclusive environments. It allows designers, owners and managers of environments, to assess the relevance to them of particular information.	Tel: 020 7944 8011 www.dptac.gov.uk
Disability Rights Commission (DRC)	Tel (helpline): 08457 622 633 www.drc-gb.org
The Disability Unit at the Department of Works and Pensions	www.disability.gov.uk
Employers' Forum on Disability	Tel: 020 7403 3020 www.employers-forum.co.uk
English Heritage	Tel: 0870 333 1181 www.english-heritage.org.uk

Foundation for Assistive Technology	Tel: 020 7253 3303 www.fastuk.org
Guide Dogs for the Blind Association (GDBA)	Tel: 0870 600 2323 www.guidedogs.org.uk
Helen Hamlyn Research Centre	Tel: 020 7590 4242 www.hhrc.rca.ac.uk
Historic Scotland	Tel: 0131 668 8600 www.historic-scotland.gov.uk
International Institute for Information Design (IIID)	www.iiid.net Tel: +43 1 403 6662
Is there an accessible loo? (ITAAL)	www.itaal.org.uk
Industry Committee for Emergency Lighting	Tel: 020 8675 5432 www.aecportico.co.uk/Directory/ICEL.shtm
JMU Access Partnership	Tel: 020 7391 2002 www.jmuaccess.org.uk
Joseph Rowntree Foundation	Tel: 01904 629241 www.jrf.org.uk
National Disability Arts Forum	Tel: 0191 261 1628 www.ndaf.org.uk
National Register of Access Consultants (NRAC)	Tel: 020 7234 0434 www.nrac.org
Office of the Deputy Prime Minister	Tel: 020 7944 4400 www.odpm.gov.uk
Research and Information for Consumers with Disabilities	Tel: 020 7427 2460 www.ricability.org.uk
Research Group for Inclusive Environments (RGIE)	Tel: 0118 378 6734 www.reading.ac.uk/ie
Royal Association of Disability and Rehabilitation (RADAR)	Tel: 020 7250 3222 www.radar.org.uk
Royal Institute of British Architects	Tel: 020 7580 5530 www.riba.org
Royal Institution of Chartered Surveyors	Tel: 0870 333 1600 www. rics.org.uk
Royal National Institute of the Blind (RNIB)	Tel: 020 7388 1266 www.rnib.org.uk

Royal National Institute for Deaf People (RNID)	Tel: 020 7296 8000 www.rnid.org.uk
Royal Town Planning Institute (RTPI)	Tel: 020 7929 9494 www.rtpi.org.uk
Sign Design Society	Tel: 01582 713556 www.signdesignsociety.co.uk
Ulster Environment and Heritage Service	Tel: 028 9054 3061 www.ehsni.gov.uk

C References and publications of interest from other sources

Author	Title	Publisher and ISBN	
Ander, G D	*Daylight Performance and Design* (2003)	John Willey & Sons Inc	**0 471 26299 4**
Barker, P, Barrick, J and Wilson, R	*Building Sight* (1995)	HMSO	**011 701 993 3**
Bright, K and Di Giulio, R	*Inclusive Buildings; designing and managing and accessible environment* (2002)	Blackwell Publishing	**0 632 05955 9**
Bright, K (editor)	*Disability: Making Buildings Accessible – Special Report* 2002 Edition	Workplacelaw network	**1 900 648 14 8**
Bright, K (editor)	*Disability: Making Buildings Accessible – Special Report* 2003 Edition	Workplacelaw network	**TBA**
Bright, K, Cook, G, and Harris, J	*Colour, Contrast and Perception* (1997)	University of Reading	**0 70491 202 3**
BSI	BS 5252 (1976), *Framework for colour co-ordination for building purposes*	BSI, London	
BSI	BS 8206 (1985), Part 2, *Code of practice for daylighting*	BSI, London	
BSI	BS 4800 (1989), *Schedule of paint colours for building purposes*	BSI, London	
BSI	BS 5266 (1999), (EN 1838 *Emergency Lighting*	BSI, London	
BSI	BS 8233 (1999), *Sound insulation and noise reduction for buildings*, Code of Practice	BSI, London	
CIBSE	Technical Memorandum 10 (1985), *The calculation of glare indices*	CIBSE, London	
CIBSE	Guide B5 (2002): *Noise and Vibration Control for HCAV*	CIBSE, London	
CIE	*Method of measuring and specifying colour rendering of light sources*	CIE Publication 13.2, 2nd Edition, CIE Vienna	
Cuttel, C	*Lighting by Design* (2003)	Architectural Press	**0 750651 130X**
International Committee for Emergency Lighting	Document 1006 (1999), *Emergency Lighting Design Guide*, 3rd Edition	ICEL, London	
ITAAL	*The ITAAL Directory of Accessible Loos in England* (2001)	ITAAL	**1 904155 00 6**
Lighting Industry Federation, Forster, R (ed)	*The Lighting Industry Federation Lamp Guide* (2003)	LIF, London	
Oxley, P	*Inclusive Transport*	Dept. For Transport	
Sawyer, A and Bright, K	*The Access Manual; auditing and managing inclusive built environments* (2003)		**1 4051 0765 0**

Society of Light and Lighting	*The Code for Lighting* (2001)	CIBSE, London
Tregenza, P and Loe, D	*The Design of Lighting* (1998)	Spon Press, London
Webber, G M B, Wright, M S and Cook, G K	*Emergency lighting and wayfinding systems for visually impaired people*, Information Paper IP 9/97 (1997)	Construction Research Communications Ltd, London